yoga myths

ALSO BY JUDITH HANSON LASATER

30 Essential Yoga Poses: For Beginning Students and Their Teachers

Living Your Yoga: Finding the Spiritual in Everyday Life

Relax and Renew: Restful Yoga for Stressful Times

Restore and Rebalance: Yoga for Deep Relaxation

What We Say Matters: Practicing Nonviolent Communication

A Year of Living Your Yoga: Daily Practices to Shape Your Life

Yoga Abs: Moving from Your Core

Yoga for Pregnancy: What Every Mom-to-Be Needs to Know

Yogabody: Anatomy, Kinesiology, and Asana

yoga myths

WHAT YOU NEED TO LEARN AND UNLEARN FOR A SAFE AND HEALTHY YOGA PRACTICE

Judith Hanson Lasater

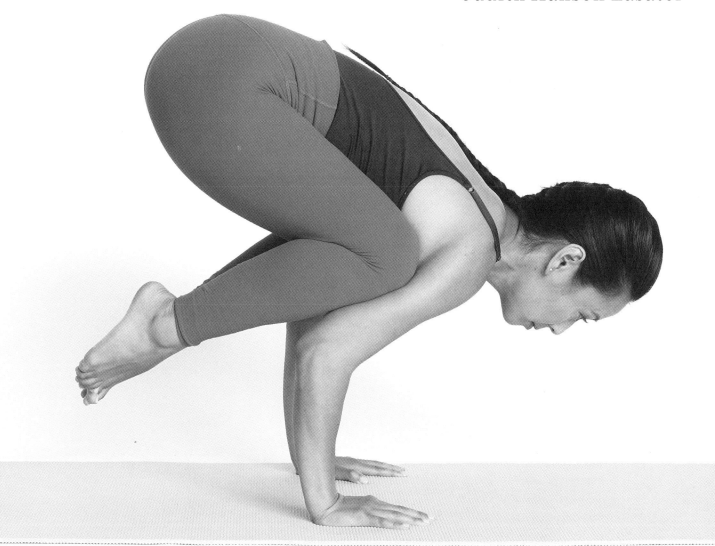

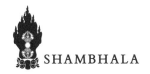

SHAMBHALA

Shambhala Publications, Inc.
4720 Walnut Street
Boulder, Colorado 80301
www.shambhala.com

Front cover photo: David Martinez
Cover design and interior design: Laura Shaw Design

9 8 7 6 5 4 3 2 1

FIRST EDITION

Printed in the United States of America

⊖ This edition is printed on acid-free paper that meets the American National
Standards Institute Z39.48 Standard.
♻ Shambhala Publications makes every effort to print on recycled paper.
For more information please visit www.shambhala.com.
Shambhala Publications is distributed worldwide by Penguin Random House, Inc.,
and its subsidiaries.

Library of Congress Cataloging-in-Publication Data

Names: Lasater, Judith, author.
Title: Yoga myths: what you need to learn and unlearn for a safe and
   healthy yoga practice / Judith Hanson Lasater.
Description: First edition. | Boulder, Colorado: Shambhala, [2020] |
   Includes bibliographical references and index.
Identifiers: LCCN 2019042112 | ISBN 9781611807967 (trade paperback)
Subjects: LCSH: Hatha yoga.
Classification: LCC RA781.7 .L376 2020 | DDC 613.7/046—dc23
LC record available at https://lccn.loc.gov/2019042112

For Glyn Elizabeth, Karen, Nico, Joe, and

all my grandchildren, with great love

Contents

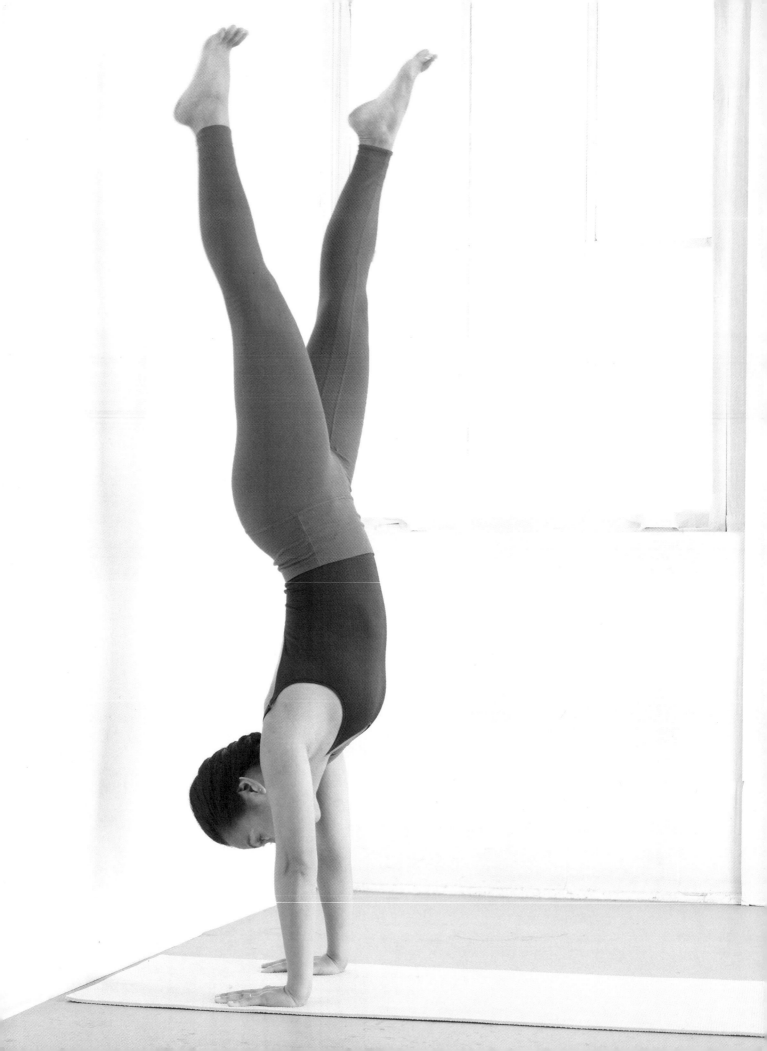

Foreword

Trust yourself first. —JUDITH HANSON LASATER

MANY OF US have heard and shared the refrain "Everything happens for a reason." While we might engage in discussion about the relevance of synchronicities and luck, dumb or otherwise, it seems likely we can agree that sometimes we experience life in a way that reveals the locus of the muted, hidden places within us. Circumstances unfold in such a way that we awaken to the impetuses behind our choices as well as the residues. Frequently, we enlist the support of a trusted teacher to guide our inquiry and help us recover our footing when it feels like the earth has fallen out from under us. If we're fortunate, we connect with someone who models a way to be in the world that resonates with our "heart brain." When I think back to September 2002, I see clearly how my decision to attend a shoulder anatomy workshop pulled me onto the path I tread today. That workshop was led by my dear teacher, mentor, colleague, and friend, Judith Hanson Lasater.

Over the course of three days, Judith shared clear, sensible descriptions of the shoulder and its movements. I felt immediate and welcome changes in the asana we practiced during her lessons. To this day, my shoulders—and the rest of me—are grateful that I went to that workshop! More than the relief provided by healthy joint positioning, this experience also left an indelible imprint on my psyche. Judith was the first yoga teacher with whom I'd studied that asked for my consent to be touched. She never exerted power over me; instead, she consistently reflected back to me my own inner wisdom by asking about my experience and inviting me to explore further. By studying anatomy and kinesiology in the context of asana, I learned to trust my body's natural intelligence and somatic awareness, a state that Judith calls "body-fulness." As a consequence of connecting to my bodyfulness, I began to trust my own inner wisdom.

The book that you look at now is a summation of Judith's decades-long practice and study of asana. *Yoga Myths* is an invitation to create asana from a foundation of trust: in our bodies, intuition, and self-awareness. The chapters that follow are also informed by her rigorous study of our form, function, and movement. Judith melds anatomical realities with her many years of teaching to thousands of students the world over. *Yoga Myths* presents a framework for practice that encourages each of us to shape asana for ourselves, guided by respect for each person's unique anatomy, healthy directions and ranges of movement, and self-compassion. Each chapter offers an opportunity to understand and explore how different movement choices in asana affect our bodily sensations as well as the feelings and emotions that accompany them. Rather than prescribing strict "alignment" principles to create asana that match externally imposed ideas of presentation, Judith invites us to see, feel, move, and trust our bodyfulness. She welcomes each of us to make informed choices from the foundation of our personal structure, shaped by our relationship with gravity, to deepen our somatic and psychic exploration of asana.

Yoga Myths is an invaluable resource for students and teachers alike. Judith's accurate and direct explanations of how we choose to express asana harken us to the inner voices that echo within our interstitial space. Now, take this book, set up your practice space, and experiment with some myth-busting on the mat.

—Mary Richards, MS
Yoga teacher and anatomy nerd
Alexandria, Virginia
November 2019

Introduction

WHAT IS A YOGA MYTH AND WHY DO YOU NEED TO KNOW?

L ET ME BEGIN with a story about my first class teaching yoga. I will then explain more about yoga myths, what they are, and why we need to educate ourselves to avoid getting stuck in believing them. At the end of this introduction, I will suggest how to use this book to guide you on your journey as you rediscover the inherent intelligence to be found in natural movement.

I remember the first yoga class I ever taught. Walking into that class, I felt naively confident. But that confidence quickly dissolved because it was based solely on the fact that I loved yoga and practiced myself every day. While this enthusiasm was a great asset, it was not enough; I had absolutely no formal training in how to teach.

This lack of training soon became apparent to me and inspired me to attend physical therapy school and to study for a PhD in East-West psychology. Even though I graduated many years ago, I still continue to study the art and craft of teaching yoga. I believe that teaching yoga is a privilege, not a right, and that the best teachers always yearn to understand more about what is safe and effective to teach, and how they can effectively communicate that to students. I also want to train my students on how to practice safely and effectively, rather than just putting them through their paces while they are in class.

Because yoga has become more and more popular and integrated into Western culture, millions of people outside of India study and practice yoga. Along with this has come a proliferation of yoga teachers.

What I have noticed almost universally when I travel to teach yoga teachers is that there are a number of commonly taught principles in yoga classes that are not based in what I call "anatomical reality." Some of these principles can interfere with the body's structure and the way the joints and muscles actually work in asana (posture or pose) practice, as well as in normal daily movement.

This observation has inspired me to write this book. My dream is to contribute to the education of yoga students and yoga teachers. I like to tell my students, "I want to teach you in a way that enables you to take a class in any style of asana practice and know how to keep yourself safe."

I know you can do more in your poses, and in your life for that matter, but my real challenge to you is can you do *less*? Alignment and ease are always more important in asana practice than an ambitious, increased, and forced range of movement. *Honoring this principle of consciously doing slightly less will go a long way toward keeping you safe and happy on your yoga mat.* And it will allow you, I believe, to continue practicing asana with pleasure through your 60s, 70s, and even for some, into your 80s and 90s.

In this book, I introduce what I call "yoga myths" in each chapter. These are the beliefs commonly held about how movements *should* be practiced, which in fact do not represent the actual physical anatomical reality of the body's structure and how it moves. These yoga myths are very common among virtually all systems of yoga asana practice.

Each chapter of this book has several parts, the first of which is an original quote from me. The next section is entitled "Why You Need to Know This." Here I offer a story from my teaching experience that reflects the importance of why I have found the major points of the chapter important and useful in practicing and teaching.

The next part, "Your Structure," explains the anatomical structure relating to the topic of the chapter in a way that is not only interesting but that also empowers you to put information to practical use. This is followed by what I consider the most important part of each chapter: "Your Anatomy in Action." It is not enough to understand some basic structural facts about how our human body is constructed. We must turn those facts into useful knowledge, understanding how the individual parts of the body actually work together when we move.

I like the analogy of an orchestra. The individual musicians create music with their instruments, but the power of that music is truly unleashed when all the instruments are played together in synchrony. Human movement is as complicated and intricate as a symphony orchestra playing together, if not more so. Each part of our structure works together to allow us to do a wide variety of things: to stand, to walk, to practice asana, to balance on our hands, to lie down and rest, and so on.

When the "orchestra" of the body is playing in a graceful and delicious flow, movement is efficient, pain free, and beautiful. If the body's natural intelligence is interrupted by injury or by an unclear intellectual belief of how movements should be created or by the lack of embodied awareness, there are always consequences.

These consequences, or limitations, are often why students seek out yoga asana practice in the first place; they have a direct experience of what happens when there is no harmony in their movement. They present themselves to their yoga teachers with headaches, mental agitation, back pain, knee pain, joint stiffness, muscle tightness, postural imbalances, digestive issues, and other organ dysfunctions, as well as the inability to lie on the floor and relax deeply and contentedly for twenty minutes.

What we, as both yoga students and teachers, need to learn is what I call "movement literacy." Just as we become literate when we learn to read books, I believe we need to learn to read our own and our students' movements. This will afford us the opportunity to understand clearly what has caused the injury or limitation, as well as the pain associated with that movement.

Then we will be able to offer to ourselves and to others a different way of inhabiting and using the body that can contribute to a deeper sense of well-being and health. When we see our students or ourselves with soft eyes, we see through the lens of truth and compassion. This helps us better understand how we, or our students, arrived at this place of dysfunction in the first place. Then we can create the opportunity to choose something different in our practice and teaching of yoga. This difference is that we now have the power to stop injuring ourselves and to begin to move with more joy and ease.

How to Use This Book

This book is certainly about information, but mostly it is about practice. My suggestion is that you read each chapter at least twice, if at all possible, to really comprehend the anatomical and movement principles that are given there.

Then I suggest you get on your mat and practice one of the poses or techniques offered in the section titled "Attentive Practice." Be sure to take your time and practice with a focus on detail and sensation. Trust yourself and what your body is telling you.

Remember that you may be trying something that is not only new, but also something that may be the *exact opposite* of what you have been taught, or what you have been practicing, or what you have been teaching. Cultivate patience and an open mind. Be curious.

I strongly suggest that if you are a teacher, you do not rush immediately to teach a new technique you have just learned. Let your new learning soak into your cells and make it your own, and then in due time it will be expressed to your students in an integrated manner.

Finally, enjoy yourself, whatever level of experience and ability you bring to your mat. Yoga practice is important but not serious. Invite the spirit of play into your learning. And remember you are in charge of you. Do just enough for today.

yoga myths

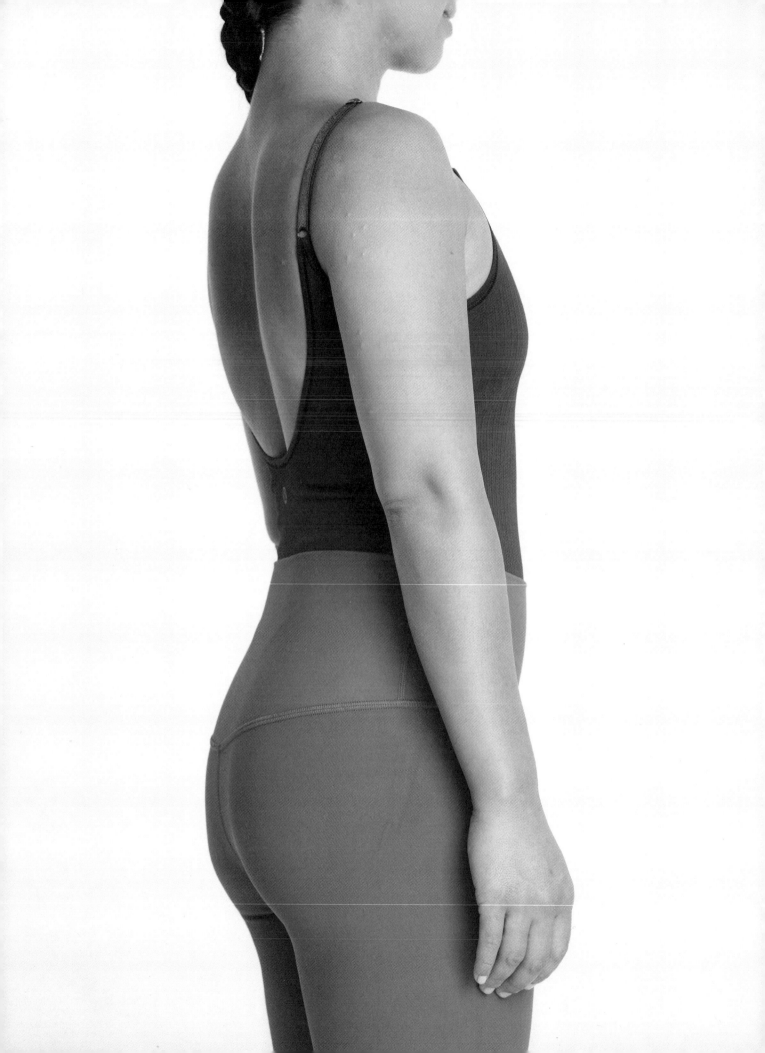

1

It's All about the Curves

STOP TUCKING YOUR TAILBONE

The normal spinal curves allow us the perfect balance between freedom of movement and the power of stability.

UNDERSTANDING WHEN to tuck and when not to tuck will change your life. I do not exaggerate. I have heard countless stories from yoga students who have said that when they learned to love their normal curves and let those curves be present in standing, not only did it reduce their pain, but it also lifted their spirits. Let me begin with one of these stories.

I will always cherish the memory of a sweet experience I had leading a class for teachers on the topic of understanding the curves of the spinal column and applying that understanding to teaching asana.

Students were invited to come up to the front of the class if they wanted to and to share their standing posture with the class in a friendly and supportive atmosphere so we could observe different body types. As one woman was showing us her pose, she related that frequently she heard from teachers that her lumbar spine (lower back) was too arched, and that she should tuck more, thus reducing the curve. She tried and tried to do this for years, but the pose never felt right and took a lot of effort to attempt to maintain this flatter column.

I asked her to stand in the way that felt the best to her. Then with her permission, I put my hands lightly on her top pelvis so that I could feel the top of the "bowl" of the pelvis and, after a couple other simple tests, concluded that her pelvis was indeed very likely in a neutral position.

In other words, she was not at all arched for her body; neither was she tucked. From my observation and palpation, she was in fact standing with *her very own neutral curve in her lower back*. This meant that she had just the right amount of lower back curve for *her body*.

When I shared this information quietly with her, tears began to roll down her face. I asked her why she was crying, and her answer was, "I feel like I have finally been given permission to be myself." All of us who witnessed this were very touched by her clarity and honesty. She had given up the yoga "myth" that her vertebral column needed to be flat and straight.

In hindsight, I realized that "being one's Self" is actually at the core of what yoga practice is all about. All the practices of yoga are about "returning" to what was already there: our inherent wisdom, our natural goodness, and our spiritual wholeness. That moment with the student mentioned above was a "yoga" moment of her remembering herself in a pure way.

I write about this story simply because this book is all about listening to your teachers but simultaneously trusting yourself in your own practice. If we just follow others' directions when we practice, it is difficult to find our own practice. But if we aren't open to experiencing something new, it is hard to learn and grow. My wish is that you find balance between these two extremes in each of your poses at home and in each class you take.

I want for us all to practice our yoga asana with intelligent and kind persistence as we uncover our own true Selves. Certainly, I also want these qualities to be applied as we discover our own individual spinal curves and their power and importance in our lives and practice.

Why You Need to Know This

Simply put, all of the human body's positions involve the vertebral column. Therefore, all asana involve the vertebral column, whether we are standing, inverted, seated, twisting, or lying down, the spinal column is at the receptive center of our body, our poses, and our entire practice.

We celebrate when a baby first learns to stand up as an important human milestone for each person. Interestingly, in asana class we often begin our practice standing in a vertical line. This asana is named Mountain Pose, or Tadasana in Sanskrit, and it helps us to bring awareness to the very same vertical line we claimed in babyhood.

Human beings stand up on two feet, and we need to do it well because poor posture can affect every system in the body, including the immune system, the respiratory system, the cardiovascular system, and the digestive system, as well as the health of our bones, the function of our muscles and our metabolism, and other normal functions.[1] Posture reflects and can greatly influence our mood, how others see and judge us, and simply how we feel about ourselves and about being alive.[2]

Modern society has by and large changed the way we use our bodies on a daily basis, in large part by shifting us toward much more sitting time and much less walking and moving around time in which we are constantly assuming different positions. One of the consequences of this shift toward less movement is an increase in the incidence of repetitive strain injuries. These types of injuries happen when we do the same movement over and over, like sitting and typing at a computer.

However, society has not significantly changed our basic human structure and how that structure functions. If we are to stay safe and happy on our yoga mat, and to enjoy our practice of yoga for all the years of our life, respect for and understanding of the function and structure of the vertebral column is crucial. This idea is based on the premise that true freedom comes from self-awareness and self-knowledge. And those principles are not just philosophical or spiritual precepts. I believe they are imbued in the body as well, and that we can feel them, understand them, and adapt to them. But first we must understand our structure and how it works.

Your Structure

One of the most remarkable things about the vertebral column is its ability to adapt to a wide variety of human postures and movements. And this is in large part due to the fact that the column is shaped into three specific curves, with the sacrum at the base that is fused into a single permanent curve and joined with the pelvis.

The first curve is the cervical curve (neck) and is made up of seven vertebrae named from the top to the bottom C1 to C7. The second curve is the thoracic curve with twelve vertebrae, T1 to T12. Each thoracic vertebra has two ribs attached. The third moveable curve is the lumbar spine, and each segment is named from L1 to L5.

The last part of the column, and the part of the spine that joins with the pelvis, is the sacrum; it fully fuses into a solid curved bone at about the age of twenty-five. Note that the cervical and lumbar

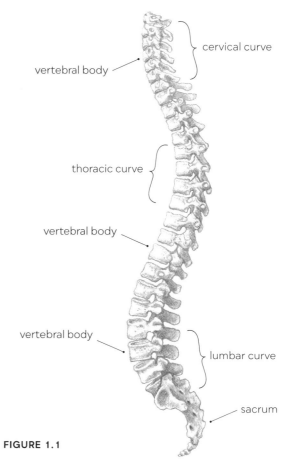

cervical curve

vertebral body

thoracic curve

vertebral body

vertebral body

lumbar curve

sacrum

FIGURE 1.1

curves are facing the same way, which is the opposite of how the thoracic and sacral curves face. So I like to think of the curves of the vertebral column like the curves of a river moving across a plain.

Between most of the vertebrae are intervertebral discs. These are a form of connective tissue and serve the purposes of bearing weight and cushioning and protecting the vertebral bodies, as well as keeping the bodies apart and thus creating space between them and contributing to a full range of movement at each segment.

The discs, which are connected to the vertebral bodies, have a softer center, the nucleus pulposus, which is surrounded by fibrous rings. This structure helps the discs bear weight more effectively and adapt to the different positions that the vertebral column assumes during the day.

Furthermore, the wedge-like shape of the discs actually helps to create the normal curves. Notice how the *anterior* aspect of the intervertebral discs in the cervical lumbar region have more height and are tapered to a shorter height *posteriorly*. In the thoracic region, the wedge shape is the opposite, with the *posterior* aspect of the discs thicker than the front. Like the cervical discs, the lumbar discs taper *posteriorly*.

Please notice, too, that the discs are located close to where the spinal nerves exit from the spinal cord. If your discs bulge or move out of place, they can press on these nerves and cause radiating nerve pain in your body, which can be debilitating.

Remember that the curves we are discussing here are considered "normal vertebral curves." There is a type of curve in the column that is called scoliosis and is not considered normal. Scoliosis is a side bending curve, and not a front to back curve like the normal curves. In scoliosis, there is also a rotational component expressed in the column.

If you suspect you may have scoliosis, please do have it checked out with a professional health-care provider. They can offer you information and exercises that may help you to improve. I do have several students and friends who manage their scoliosis well with yoga practice.

The two main functions of the spinal curves are to allow for efficient movement and to provide maximum stability when needed. Some people find it counterintuitive that a curve, like a column, can be stable. All around us we see stable buildings that are designed and constructed in straight lines. I live in earthquake country, and if I were in a building with curved walls, I would likely be uneasy in that structure, as I would doubt its stability.

The paradox with the body is that the curved anatomy of the vertebral bodies and the wedge-shaped discs create congruence at each spinal segment. This means that when the curves are in their neutral state, that is, curved just enough, it creates the body's most stable "line" because there is maximum surface area touching at each vertebral segment through the discs and bodies of the vertebrae. In the field of gravity, holding your spine in a straight line is not the most stable position for the column, regardless of what you might think.

But the curved stability of the column is not just produced by the bodies of the vertebrae and the discs. The vertebrae join through their bodies and discs in the front, and they also join at the back. On the posterior side of each vertebra are two structures at the lower end and two at the upper end called facets.

On each vertebra, these flattened facet surfaces join together flattened surfaces on the vertebrae above and below it to create a facet joint. This is like two halves of a doughnut put together to make a whole doughnut. A single facet joins with another single facet to make a whole joint. Remember that a joint is defined as the place where two bones come together.

The effect is a whole series of facet joints on either side of the column, from top to bottom, and with the anterior bodies, they create a kind of "tripod stool" at each individual segment. The facets form two "legs," and the bodies and discs together create the third "leg" of the tripod weight-bearing "stool." When this happens, you will be maximally stable in your vertebral column when standing.

When the three legs of the stool are congruent, the force of gravity will be borne well by the bones of your spinal column, and thus you will be held upright with minimal effort required from your muscles. Standing in the natural curves will also be less stressful for your soft tissues, like ligaments and tendons, because there will be maximum stability at each segment and the bones will be supporting your weight well.

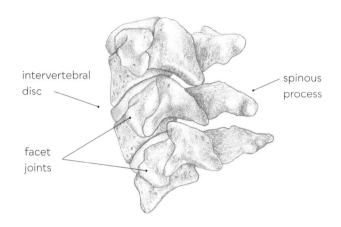

intervertebral disc

spinous process

facet joints

FIGURE 1.2

Your Anatomy in Action

Note to the reader: Please be mindful of your body when attempting the simple movements suggested in this section of the chapter. Do take into account any limitation or injuries you may have in your spinal column, and if you are unsure about whether to try them, then don't. You may want to consult your health-care practitioner before beginning your practice, as well as an experienced yoga teacher.

The principle to understand in this chapter is that the spinal curves are normal and functional in the vertebral column. Straightening or flattening the column in Mountain Pose, while intellectually satisfying perhaps, is like asking someone to stand on a tripod stool with only one leg on the ground. In this case, the "one leg" is at the front of the spine: the bodies of the vertebrae and their intervertebral discs. In flexion of the column, the posterior side opens and thus the facets are partially disengaged, making this connection less stable.

When you bend forward or backward, or rotate your vertebral column, you distort your curves. This is how we move, and it is healthy and normal. What can become problematic is when we habitually distort our spinal curves, as when we carry our head in a forward posture most of the time. This distorted position of the neck greatly increases the load the neck structures must carry in order to keep the head up against gravity.

Getting stuck in any posture in which the normal curves are distorted is problematic for the soft tissues like discs, fascia (connective tissue), and muscles. The neck is especially susceptible to stress when the cervical spine is distorted in standing by being positioned ahead of the body.

This is much more likely to happen when you tuck your pelvis in Mountain Pose because the column functions as a connected whole. According to A. I. Kapandji in *The Physiology of the Joints*, "For every inch of a Forward Head

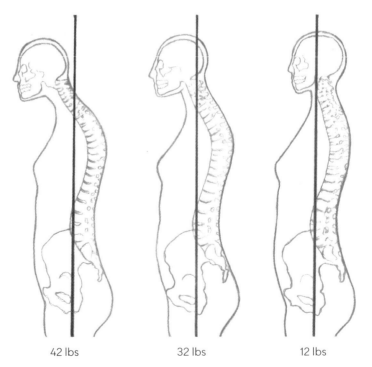

42 lbs   32 lbs   12 lbs

FIGURE 1.3
How heavy is your head?

Posture, it can increase the weight of the head on the spine by an additional 10 pounds."[3]

Sometimes students who are tucking the pelvis compensate by lifting the sternum (breastbone), an action that flattens the thoracic curve. This will bring the head back over the body but at the cost of flattening the cervical curve. Now all the curves are distorted.

The constancy of this distortion can eventually involve dysfunction of the nerves in the form of nerve compression and pain, not to mention muscular tension and pain as well. Some people with a forward head posture complain of headaches and chronic pain in the trapezius muscle at the very top of the shoulder where you might carry a shoulder bag. Notice how you hold your head and neck when typing at the computer and when driving. Likely your head is forward—not directly over your body—and not in a normal cervical curve.

There can also be pain that is created from the strain the ligaments, fascia, and tendons (soft tissue) experience in the area. Remember, problems don't come from just holding your head forward of your body as part of a movement; they come from maintaining this forward head posture habitually. For some people, misaligned posture has been present for as long as years and even for decades.

What forward head posture consists of is actually a forward bend or flattening of the lower cervical curve from joints C3 to C7 and a simultaneous backbending of the upper cervical curve at joints at the skull and C1 and between the C1 and C2 vertebrae.

Try this if your neck will allow: Sit well on a firm chair with a natural curve in your lower back. Make sure you are not tilting your pelvis backward. If you can feel your ischial tuberosities (sitting bones) on the chair, it will help. You should be sitting slightly forward of the sitting bones. If you feel your weight behind your sitting bones, and more on the soft tissue of the buttocks, you are very likely in flexion and not in a normal lumbar curve.

When you sit well, you will find that your head is naturally over your body. Now lower your head about halfway down, so you are looking about a foot in front of you. Keeping your neck forward, just roll your skull backward so you are backbending the upper neck to bring your eyes parallel to the horizon. You can do this by jutting your chin out. You will now notice that your head is well ahead of your body. You will also notice that you have disturbed both your thoracic and lumbar curves. Ideally, find a head position in which the outer curve of your ear is positioned in a direct vertical line over your shoulder. Notice how creating this position creates ripple effects: not only has your head position changed, but the rest of your vertebral column has adapted as well.

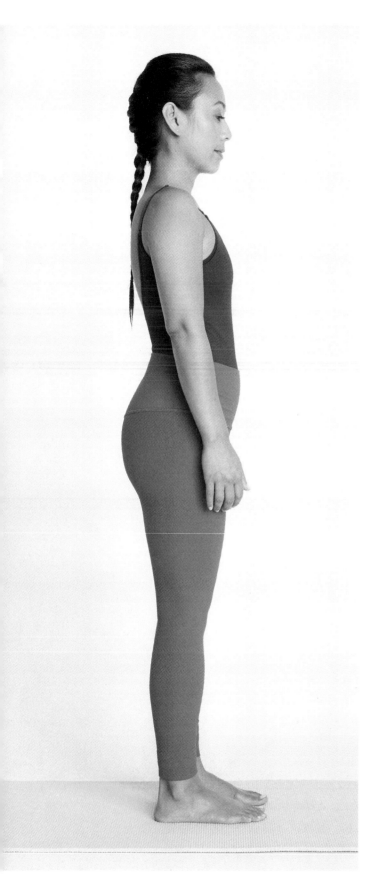

FIGURE 1.4

Distorting the lumbar curve by "tucking the tailbone" in standing is just as problematic for the lumbosacral spine as the forward head posture is for the neck. This instruction to tuck the tailbone is more often than not insisted upon in many yoga classes, especially in the vertical standing posture, Mountain Pose.

A very small percentage of people stand with too much lumbar curve, with an anterior tilt of the pelvis. But in the many decades of teaching on six continents, I have found it to be overwhelmingly true that in Western countries, although not exclusively so, modern culture tends toward a tucked pelvis due to the prevalence of sitting.

However, occasionally, a student does display too much lumbar curve, which is also a difficult posture to maintain. Typically, the individual will feel a pinching sensation from their mid- to lower lumbar region. This individual needs to pull the ASIS (anterior superior iliac spine) upward, or slightly tuck.

How can you tell if you or your student is standing in neutral? This can be difficult unless you have been specifically trained on how to ascertain this. It is easy to be fooled by the flesh of the buttocks and how the body appears from the side and back in general. If you are unsure of whether you have too much lumbar curve, consult with a trained professional or two to get their opinions. Sometimes even doctors or physical therapists can miss this one.

Sometimes you hear yoga teachers say "drop the sacrum," or "lengthen the tailbone (coccyx)." This is what I call "sneaky tucking." If you pay attention, attempting to follow either of these instructions, or similar ones, can only happen when you flex, or flatten, your lumbar spine.

When you do this, you not only destabilize your lumbar spine, but very significantly, you destabilize the joint between your sacrum and your ilia, the pair of large bones of the pelvis.

With the normal curves intact (see figure 1.4), the sacrum at rest is at about a 30° angle from the vertical. Let me reiterate: this average 30° angle is the *normal angle for the sacrum at rest*. The sacrum is *not* a vertical bone in neutral spinal alignment.

If your sacrum, or your student's sacrum, is vertical in Mountain Pose, the likelihood is high that the student is tucking. Do not be fooled by the apparent angle of the sacrum or the shape of the buttocks. A vertical sacrum is no longer fully congruent with the ilium and is less stable. Thus, tucking the tailbone does *not* create a more stable spine; it creates a less stable one! And since most of us sit too much anyway, we do not need to tuck our tailbones in yoga class as well; we need to come back to our natural physical intelligence of standing with normal curves.

There are other disadvantages to standing and sitting in a tucked or flexed position. When you tuck your tailbone in Mountain Pose, the incumbent weight of the trunk falls on the front leg of the "tripod," i.e., the body of the vertebrae, thus compressing the intervertebral discs, especially in the lumbar spine. The front of your body shortens.

Not only is this especially problematic for those who already have compromised discs, but it can also contribute to poor disc health in everyone. When the discs are compressed, the bodies of the vertebrae are closer together and push the discs out in a posterolateral direction.

This compression is not a problem for short periods of time, but when this process happens for long periods, like sitting for hours daily over years of your life, the discs can be permanently affected. And they can move in a posterolateral direction to press on the spinal nerves as they exit the column, causing radiating pain, muscle spasms, and potential muscle weakness.

Not only are the discs seriously impacted by consistent tucking, when we tuck our pelvis, we also affect the deep pelvic organs. With a normal curve, the downward weight of the viscera in the pelvis falls naturally backward slightly against the bodies of L4 and L5 vertebrae, therefore helping to hold these vertebrae in place. Tucking the tailbone and flattening the lower back interferes with this process. Additionally, when we stand with a flat lower back, this organ weight now falls directly down onto the pelvic floor. This can weaken the pelvic floor muscles. The downward force of the organs in a direct vertical line now also puts weight on the bladder and the uterus or prostate.

It has been suggested that this constant distortion of the cells of these organs could affect the integrity of the cell membrane, and thus the function of these cells could be altered.[4] Perhaps this habitual flat-back posture, both in sitting and standing, could contribute to prolapse of the bladder and uterus and to the generalized malfunction of these organs, as well as to the malfunction of the prostate gland.

Tucking does not just affect the organs, the neck, and the lower back in isolation. All of this goes together. The vertebral column has something called sympathetic curves. Because the cervical spine and the lumbar spine have curves that face the same way, they move in harmony.

Try this: Sit or stand with your normal curves. Now look up at the ceiling. Notice that your neck is backbending. But so is your lower back. Try it the other way. Forward bend slightly from the lower back, and you will notice the tendency of the neck to bend forward as well. This is the sympathetic action of the curves. They move in the same way.

So tucking your tailbone flattens your neck; backbending your lumbar spine also backbends your neck. Regardless of which part of your column you bend forward first, the other parts will follow the cervical and lumbar spine dance together. Another reason to stop tucking your tailbone: it might just save your neck as well.

MAIN POINTS TO REMEMBER FROM THIS CHAPTER

→ The spinal column is most stable in standing and sitting when all the natural curves are intact.

→ Stop tucking your tailbones.

→ Moving any part of your spine affects all its other parts.

Attentive Practice

Now it is time to integrate all that you have learned into your yoga practice. Read the cautions and all instructions carefully as you begin.

CAUTIONS

There are minimal cautions for practicing the poses in this section. However, be sure you are moving slowly in Cat-Cow and coordinating those movements with your breath. This will feel good and keep you in touch with what you are doing. Staying with your breath helps you prevent injury in all of the poses.

PROPS NEEDED

- Nonslip yoga mat
- Sturdy chair
- Folded yoga blanket, preferably made of cotton
- A doorway

Mountain Pose
TADASANA

To practice Mountain Pose, unroll your yoga mat on a flat surface. Experiment first with the distance of your feet. Place your feet completely together. Notice that you may feel a little less stable, and that you are likely swaying a bit. The energy in your body seems to be moving upward. It may feel difficult to be aware of the balance of your natural downward energy with the feet too close together.

Place your feet purposely too wide apart. Now it may feel like your energy and awareness can go downward easily, and you may feel connected with the earth. But it is harder to feel the upward energy.

I suggest you place your feet hip-width apart, so your feet are directly under your hip joints. Notice again the model in figure 1.4. The feet are shown as being directly under the sockets of the hips, and if you are practicing this way, you likely feel equally the energy move downward through the legs, as well as upward toward the heart.

Arrange the feet so that the outer border of the foot on the little toe side is exactly parallel with the edge of your mat or with the walls of the room. You may feel that you are standing in a pigeon-toed posture and that your knees are turning inward, but you are probably in neutral alignment with your hips and knees for the first time in Mountain Pose, and this may feel strange. (More on the alignment of hips and knees in chapter 6.)

Remember that the name of the posture is Mountain Pose. A mountain is rooted solidly in the earth, equally and simultaneously it is reaching and yearning for the heavens. When you stand well on your legs, you will not only feel more stable but also more present, quieter, less distracted, and more connected with yourself and your environment.

Now move slightly backward from your top thighs. If this makes you feel taller, you were probably tucking. Make sure your thighs are slightly rotating inward.

Take a moment at this time to take a deep breath. This should feel totally free, with no impediment. If you slightly tuck now, or slightly shift your pelvis forward and try to breathe, you will find your inhalation is inhibited by your posture. The diaphragm is connected to the L1 vertebra. When we flatten the lumbar spine in tucking, we interfere with the excursion of the diaphragm and thus with the flow of respiration.

With your tailbone tucked or with your top thighs slightly pushed forward as in figure 1.5, notice your pelvic floor.

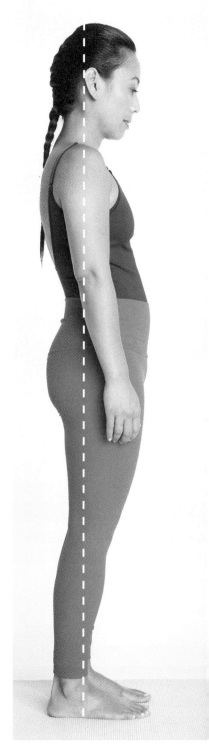

FIGURE 1.5

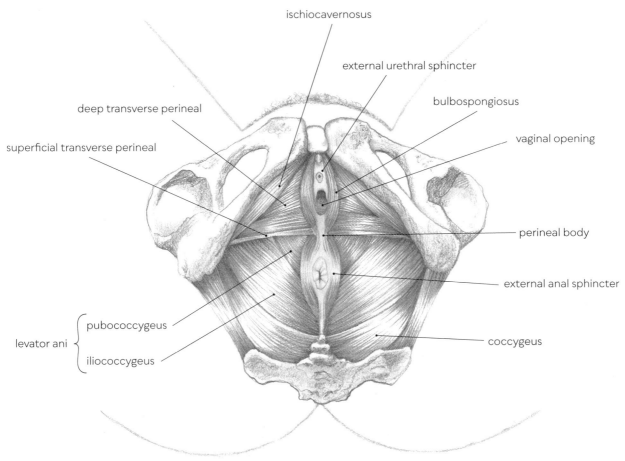

ischiocavernosus

external urethral sphincter

bulbospongiosus

deep transverse perineal

vaginal opening

superficial transverse perineal

perineal body

external anal sphincter

pubococcygeus

coccygeus

levator ani

iliococcygeus

FIGURE 1.6

The pelvic floor muscles run from the pubic bone to the coccyx and between the ischial tuberosities. This is the floor of your pelvis. You will likely feel that these muscles are sagging. It feels like the coccyx is pushing forward, and the back half of the pelvic floor muscles are collapsing forward.

Now bring your top thighs backward and notice that the pelvic floor now has its natural space and has spontaneously lifted upward, giving support to the pelvic organs. There is a sense that the pelvic floor is not inhibited, and thus it will assume its most effective shape. I believe this spontaneous upward movement of the pelvic floor is what is called in yoga *mula bandha*, or the root lock.

I do not believe that mula bandha is something that has to be practiced with a clinching effort; rather it is spontaneously created from the alignment of the legs, pelvis, and vertebral column. Mula bandha is a technique for preventing the loss of energy from the bottom of the trunk, keeping it in the body in order for it to be used for a spiritual purpose.

One of the reasons we are told to tuck the tailbone is that many people believe that it strengthens the core, the abdominal muscles. This is actually not what happens at all. When you tuck and move the thighs forward, the abdominals actually do less, not more. Tuck your tailbone, push your top thighs forward, and notice your abdomen let go. Without moving your spine or rib cage, try to contract your abdominals. You simply cannot.

Now stand in Mountain Pose with your top thighs slightly back, your pelvic floor completely free, and your uppermost legs slightly turned inward. As you move backward with your top thighs, you will notice the abdominals spontaneously contract slightly, especially the oblique abdominals that you can feel at the outer front side pelvis.

To feel this, try these two positions with your hands around your waist. Start in a tucked position and move backward from the top of the thighs. You will feel your abdominal muscles jump into action without any prompting from your mind. Your abdominals are smarter than you. They know when and how to respond to gravity in standing and will always use an appropriate amount of action to stabilize your pelvis and spinal column.

This abdominal action is not something that you have to think about doing; this is not something that you consciously create. Rather this is the natural intelligence of your body responding to perfect alignment *with* gravity. When we tuck, we are instead standing in a way that fights gravity.

Please move your attention now to your scapulae (shoulder blades). In Mountain Pose the shoulder blades need to be vertical. Notice that when you slump or tuck, your shoulder blades are resting against your back in an angle. Moving the shoulder blades into a vertical position also greatly helps to bring the head and neck into alignment.

You may want your yoga teacher or a friend to look at your shoulder blades from the side while you are standing in Mountain Pose. They can give you feedback as to whether the shoulder blades appear perpendicular. You can also notice this yourself by exaggerating a slouch when standing; feel how your shoulder blades move toward the side of your trunk and are no longer vertical. Be sure you do not overcompensate by pushing the bottom, or inferior angle, of your shoulder blades forward too much.

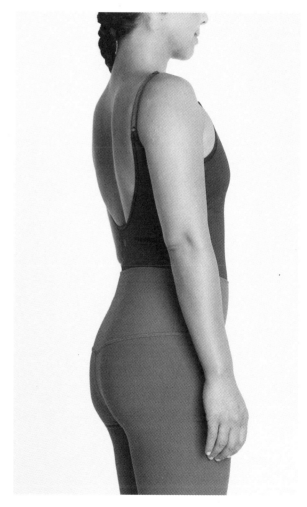

FIGURE 1.7

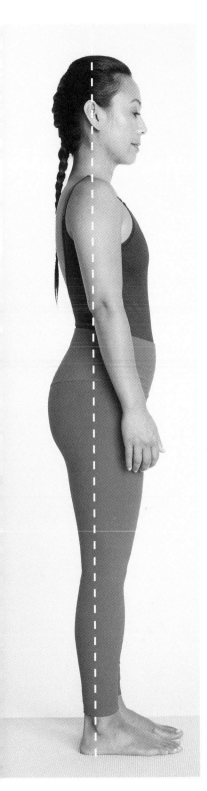

FIGURE 1.8

The sternum in Mountain Pose is also at an angle. The lowest part of the breastbone is farther away from the trunk than the upper breastbone. If we tuck the pelvis, the sternum becomes vertical and breathing is impeded. Let your arms hang naturally at your sides.

With a natural alignment the head and neck should now be poised perfectly over the body. If someone looks at you from the side, your ear opening, i.e., the external auditory meatus, will be exactly in line with the middle of the head of the humerus (upper arm bone) at the top of the side shoulder.

If this imaginary line continues downward, it will pass exactly through the middle of your side hip and anterior to the midline of the side knee and the lateral malleolus (outer anklebone). To complete the pose, slightly drop your chin so that your eyes are parallel to the horizon. Then turn your eyes slightly down themselves so they rest softly on the lower eyelids.

Bring your attention to your heart in the left center of your chest. Imagine the front heart opening but do not actually move your rib cage. Now open the back of your heart. Now open the sides of the heart. Open the ceiling of your heart and receive all blessings. At last open the floor of your heart and flood yourself with those blessings.

Move your focus to the exact center of your brain. Notice which of the two hemispheres of your brain might seem fuller than the other one. Then like a balloon, let the "air" out of the bigger hemisphere and sense the two sides of your brain as equally full, equally empty, equally floating.

It may now be hard to determine whether the act of aligning your body has created this mind state, or your mind state has created the perfect alignment of your body. It is as if you are standing in the metaphorical center of consciousness. Part of you is living completely in your body, part of you is living in the sweetness of your heart, and part of you is living in the spacious silence of your mind, all at the same time. This is Mountain Pose.

Practice this pose on your yoga mat at home, in class, and whenever you are standing in line waiting. Just thirty seconds to one minute is enough to remind you of the natural perfection of your spinal curves and of the inner meditative state of yoga.

Mountain Pose 2
ALIGNING WITH THE CORNER OF THE DOOR

Whenever you remember it in your day, practice Mountain Pose in the corner of a door.

Find a doorway and turn your back to one of the corners. Place your feet as we did in Mountain Pose above, with the outside borders of your feel parallel to the edge of your imaginary mat.

Place your coccyx bone, your mid-thoracic spine, and the back of your head against the slightly sharp edge of the door. You may have to experiment with the distance your heels are from the door. It depends on your body shape and especially the depth of your rib cage and the size of your buttocks. Make sure that your chin is exactly parallel to the floor. Most people have a tendency to lift the chin in this situation. Perhaps a friend or teacher could give you feedback on your head position. Stand here for a few breaths. Repeat this throughout the day to remind you of Mountain Pose.

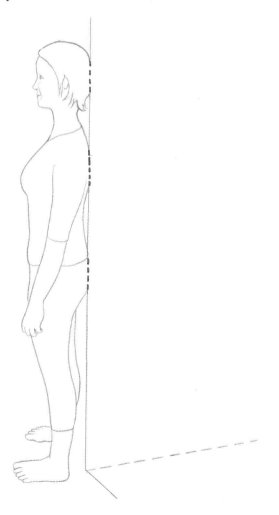

FIGURE 1.9
Mountain Pose in a doorway

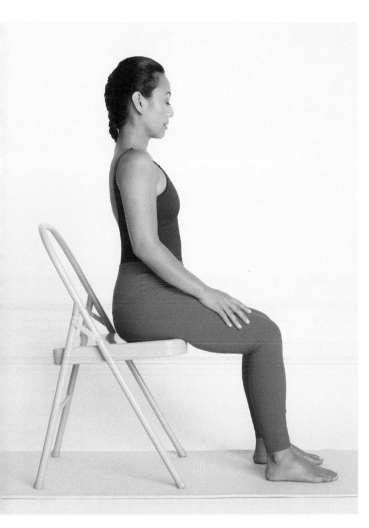

FIGURE 1.10

Mountain Pose 3

WHILE SITTING WELL

Since we sit so much, be aware of your spinal curves in sitting. The base in sitting is the pelvis and not the feet, of course, but you can build a Mountain Pose from the pelvis as well.

Remember to roll your pubic bone down so that your pelvis is exactly in the middle and not tipping back or forward. Sit slightly forward of your sitting bones. If you are working, make sure that you bring your computer and/or desktop toward you and not the other way around. Check that your head is over your body, your shoulders are dropped and shoulder blades are vertical, your breathing is unimpeded, and you feel at ease in your body and mind. It never hurts to relax your jaw as well.

Try to sit in Mountain Pose as often as you can: at your desk, at lunch (this will facilitate digestion and elimination), in your car, when meditating, and at all other times. Your breathing, digestion, thinking, and mood will be better.

Cat-Cow Pose

While these movements do not have specific Sanskrit names, they are part of other poses. The Cat portion of rounding up is part of sitting back to Hero Pose (Virasana), and the Cow portion is part of coming into Upward-Facing Dog Pose (Urdhva Adho Mukha Svanasana). These positions are useful ones to relieve your back and to help you to feel and thus to understand the sympathetic curves in your back. Practice Cat-Cow by unrolling your mat and getting down on all fours.

Drop your head and take a few breaths. Notice that when you drop your head, you instantly become more introverted. Inhale, and as you exhale, slowly begin to round your back by lifting your belly toward your back and

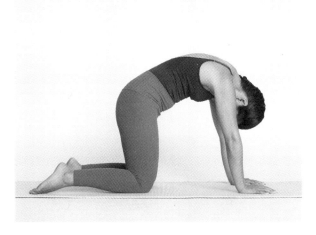

FIGURE 1.11

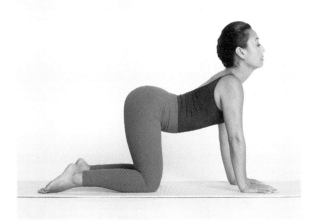

FIGURE 1.12

tucking your chin and tailbone under. Your back should look like a cat's rounded back. Be sure to tuck your chin. This is flexion of the entire column.

Now slowly let your abdomen drop below your ribs and groin as you inhale so your whole back becomes arched, with tailbone up and your neck in a backbend in Cow Pose.

Repeat these two positions slowly six to eight times. Make sure to coordinate your breathing with the movements.

To feel the sympathetic curves, let the movement begin in the center abdomen as above, but this time try to use each part of your back in a sequential way, vertebra by vertebra, so the tailbone and the head at the far ends are the very last to move into flexion.

Reverse the process now so that only the middle of your body is moving into a backbend and the ends of the column and the pelvis are still curled under. Move slowly so that you feel the moment when each segment is reversing from flexion to backbended spine.

Inhale as you move into the backbend. When the backbend is complete, your spinal column is in extension. Notice that as soon as the lumbar spine begins to extend, so does the neck, and vice versa. Repeat this for six to eight times. It usually feels wonderful on your lower back. Use this practice as a warm-up for other yoga poses or at the end of your asana practice before you lie down for Deep Relaxation Pose (Savasana), also known as Corpse Pose.

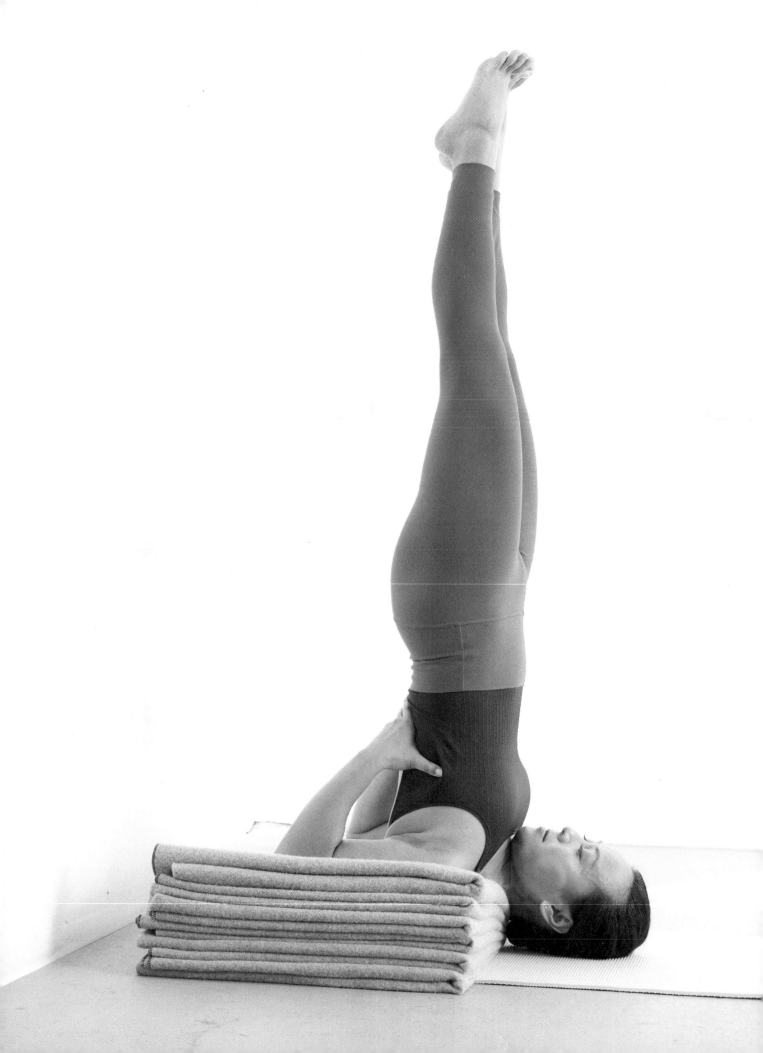

2

Saving Your Neck

WHY YOU DON'T NEED NECK ROLLS BUT DO NEED
BLANKETS FOR SHOULDER STAND

When standing, the posture of the neck reflects the posture of the spinal column below it.

I USED TO PRACTICE neck rolls constantly, whether I was practicing yoga asana or not. I was all about "cracking" my neck by moving it around in various directions. I remember once that the person sitting behind me in a movie theater actually leaned forward and asked me to stop rolling my neck around so much as it was distracting him from being able to enjoy the film. All these neck rolls were meant to "relieve" tension in my neck, and yet I still had a lingering sense of neck tension most of the time.

When I began to study with B. K. S. Iyengar in 1974, he was the first yoga teacher I had encountered who explicitly did not teach neck rolls. After a very short time of following his style of practice, my neck felt much better, and I found that I had spontaneously and slowly given up neck rolls. It was only later, when I was in physical therapy school and studying anatomy intensely, that I understood why traditional yoga asana neck rolls are nonfunctional movements for the cervical spine.

My next epiphany about my neck was when I began to use blankets to lift and support my shoulders in Supported Shoulder Stand (Salamba Sarvangasana). When I began my practice of asana, we did Shoulder Stand flat on the floor with only a thin mat or small rug under the head and shoulders. It didn't feel that great, but I was young and adaptable, so there were no immediate untoward repercussions. I did, however, develop a callous on the skin at the level of C7, the last of the cervical vertebrae. But we all had a callous in those days, and so I thought nothing of it.

The first time I was introduced to the idea of using blankets to lift and support my shoulders, it felt very scary. I was higher up now in the pose; I felt like my chest was very open, all the way to my clavicles (collarbones) and that my legs were floating.

While this was pleasurable in most ways, it was so light and so unfamiliar that I was a little afraid of this much ease. I didn't trust it. It took me several times of practicing with blankets until I found my center in the pose. Then I had a sweetly profound experience of stillness that I had never experienced before in the pose when I practiced without blankets. But I had felt the absolute advantage of using blankets in Shoulder Stand.

Why You Need to Know This

Since my first experience with blankets, I have always practiced with as well as taught, the use of blankets in Shoulder Stand, as a technique for making the pose easier but also as a way to prevent neck injury during the pose, and to avoid the deleterious cumulative effects of years of practicing this pose flat on the floor.

But to really understand why blankets are so necessary, and why neck rolls are not, it is first important to understand how the structure of the cervical spine is shaped and how it functions in our body and in our practice. While we can practice Shoulder Stand on a flat surface, it is actually a yoga myth that this way of practicing is safe for the cervical spine. It is a yoga myth that the neck can even actually roll like the hip or shoulder joint.

As was discussed in chapter 1, the most stable position for the cervical spine is when the natural curve of the neck is respected and allowed, especially in standing and sitting. A flattened cervical curve is often caused by the habitual posture of carrying the head forward of the body, or by an injury to the neck. Anyone suffering from this can tell you that a flat cervical spine is not comfortable or preferable and does not function well.

Remember, it is not the occasional flattening of the cervical curve during the normal movements of daily activities that is problematic. Rather it is the constant flattening of the cervical spine over years and decades that can eventually lead to a permanently straight neck and its accompanying problems: headaches, facial pain, nerve pain in the arms, and a limited range of movement in the neck and shoulders.

As practitioners of yoga asana, we want to be confident that the way we are practicing is in harmony with our natural structure, and that we are not practicing either Shoulder Stand or neck movements like neck rolls that can potentially harm us over many years spent on the mat. One way to do that is to understand how the cervical spine is shaped and how it moves. This knowledge gives us solid footing for practicing and teaching.

Your Structure

The cervical spine consists of seven vertebrae that form a curve when the neck is in neutral. Most cervical vertebrae join in the front of the neck at their bodies and at the intervertebral discs. The first cervical vertebra, however, does not have a body. The fused remnants of the atlas body have become part of C2 to form the odontoid process, or dens.

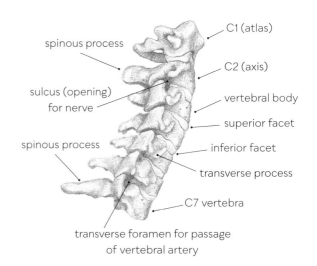

FIGURE 2.1

As mentioned in chapter 1, the cervical vertebral bodies also join together at two flattened bony surfaces on the back of the vertebrae called a facet. When the superior facet surfaces of one vertebra join with the inferior joint surfaces of the vertebral body below it, a facet joint is formed.

Each highly moveable region of the vertebral column, be it cervical, thoracic, or lumbar, has a different angle of facet surfaces. This means the angle where the two surfaces of the cervical facets connect is distinct from the thoracic facets, which are in turn distinct from the lumbar facets. (The sacral facet surfaces join only with the fifth lumbar vertebrae.)

Remember, it is this angle where the facet joints interface that determines what movements are feasible and desirable in each region of the column, and these angles are quite different region to region.

As can be seen in figure 2.1 above, in the cervical spine, these angles are at about 45° when observed from the side. The top two cervical vertebrae, C1 and C2, have some notable exceptions in their facet surfaces, but the majority of the cervical facets are similar.

What does this particular angle of 45° of the cervical facets tell us about what movements are possible for the neck? The anatomical answer to this question will clarify why neck rolls are not a great idea.

Your Anatomy in Action

To understand the principle that the angle of the facet joints predicts and thus allows very specific movement, closely study the cervical facets from the side. Note again the angle of the facet surfaces.

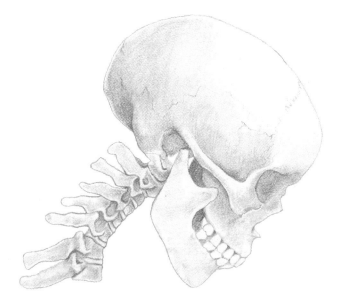

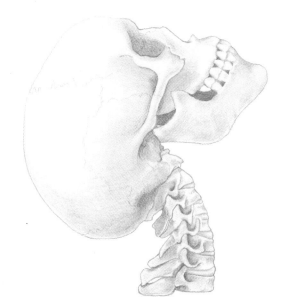

FIGURE 2.2
Cervical flexion—facets move forward and up

FIGURE 2.3
Cervical extension—facets move down and back

When you move your neck into flexion by dropping your chin down, you are moving the facets forward and up, thus the phrase "forward and up" is another way of saying "flexion."

When you flex your cervical spine, you put more pressure on the anterior structures of the vertebrae, the body and the intervertebral discs. The facets are now opening posteriorly and are bearing less weight than they do in a vertical position. In flexion, the weight is transferred forward more onto the cervical intervertebral discs.

When you extend the cervical spine, the facets move down and back, and this movement is what happens when you extend, or backbend. You do this with your neck when you lift your chin and bend backward with your neck.

Be sure you are not just moving your head forward, jutting your chin out to look up. Rather, be sure you are actually taking your whole neck and head backward. Be careful as you do this and only try a small movement if that feels better to you.

Thus when you look down, the facets open in the back and put weight on the front structures like the intervertebral discs. When you look up and back, the facets are sliding down and back on each, taking weight off the front structures and placing it on the posterior side so that it is more on the facets. This is a little like the closing of a telescope.

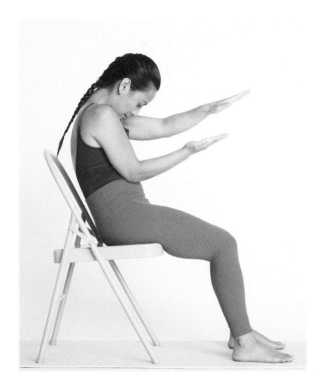

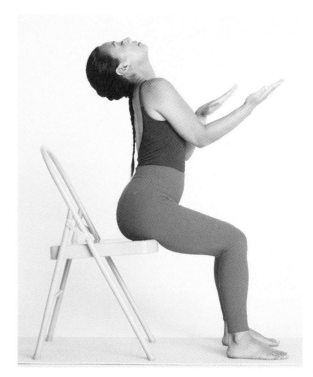

FIGURE 2.4   FIGURE 2.5

To understand this, hold your hands out in front. Turn your left palm down and your right palm up. Keep your right palm still, and slide your left hand forward and up. This movement is what the facet surfaces do when we move into flexion, or forward bending. It might help you feel this if you move your neck into flexion at the same time.

Now try the opposite; slide your left hand down and back away from the right palm. This movement is what the facet surfaces do in extension, or backbending. Backbend your neck simultaneously. This movement opens all the anterior structures of the column.

Here is the most interesting thing about understanding the movement of forward and up (flexion) and the movement of down and back (extension) in the facet joints: this is all the cervical facets can do.

You read correctly. *This is all the cervical facets can do.* But what about cervical rotation? you might ask. You certainly rotate your neck to look over your shoulder whenever you want to see behind you. How does this happen if there is only flexion and extension in the cervical spine?

In order to rotate your neck to the right, for example, the facet joints on the right move down and back (backbend) and the facet joints on the left move forward and up (forward bend). When this happens, rotation is easy. If one of your facet joints is not sitting correctly, when you try to rotate your

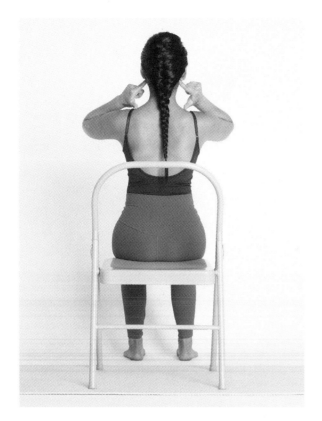

FIGURE 2.6

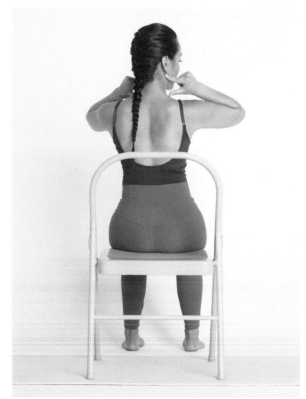

FIGURE 2.7

neck, you will probably feel a "stuck" place and/or discomfort or even pain. This is because the kinetic chain of the cervical spine has a segment or two that is not moving as it should.

Try this. Sit tall in a chair, with all your spinal curves in neutral. Take care to have all your spinal curves intact. In other words, don't round your lower back or your thoracic area. Your head should now be directly over your body, with your eyes and chin parallel to the floor. Place your right thumb on the side of your neck at the exact point your neck meets the top of your trunk. Now stretch your right index finger upward so it presses on your neck just below the ear lobe. Do the same with your left hand. Your palms will be facing toward your body.

Keeping your fingers pressed firmly to your neck and head, slowly turn your head to the right. Do not force the rotation, be comfortable in your movement and keep the chin parallel to the floor during the movement. You will notice that the fingers on the right side of your neck physically become closer together, and your left fingers are moved farther apart. This is because when you turn to the right, the right side of your neck is actually becoming shorter and the left side is actually becoming longer.

Turn your head to the left and notice the opposite occurring. Now try turning from right to left and left to right slowly back and forth without stopping.

Use a moderate speed. It becomes easily apparent that the neck is backbending (extending) on the short side and forward bending (flexing) on the long side at the same time.

With extension, the down-and-back position, the facets are packed closer together like the cylinders of a telescope when you close it. When you open the cylinders, the telescope gets longer. This is what is happening with flexion: the forward-and-up movement opens the facets like opening the cylinders of a telescope.

The neck is also capable of coupled movements. While all the cervical facets can do is to move forward and up (flexion) and down and back (extension), the results of that ability can be varied by which muscles are involved. The joints do the same thing; the muscles called upon are different. Because different muscles are acting, the end result may be flexion, extension, rotation, side bending, or some combination thereof, but in the joints the action is simply just forward and up and down and back.

If this is clear to you, then it becomes clear why neck rolls do not follow the natural intelligence of the cervical spine. The facet surfaces are very slightly curved but look almost flat. The cervical facet joints are not ball-and-socket joints.

We can move our hip joints, for example, in a circular motion because they are certainly ball-and-socket joints. But to create a neck roll we treat nonball-and-socket joints, the cervical facets, like they are ball-and-socket joints when they are actually plane, or gliding joints. During the process of the neck roll we are asking the cervical spine to do something it was not designed to do. This can cause discomfort and potential soft-tissue problems.

I respectfully suggest that you experiment with giving up neck rolls and see what results. In the "Attentive Practice" section of this chapter, I will offer you some simple neck movements that will stretch out a tight neck while honoring the innate structure of the body.

The second pose I want you to "see through the eyes" of the cervical spine is Shoulder Stand. There are major reasons to respect the intelligence of the cervical spine in this commonly taught asana as we shall see below.

Generally, this pose is practiced with the student's neck virtually flat on the mat, in cervical flexion, and with the lower cervical spine resting directly on a hard surface. It is very common to see students with their sternum dropping down, the chest caving in, and the weight of the body borne on the neck while they are up in the pose.

It is interesting that this pose is called Shoulder Stand when many people do the pose while actually resting on their neck. Let's explore why this typical position is not healthy for the neck and what can be done to protect the neck while actually learning to enjoy the pose more. In order to understand this

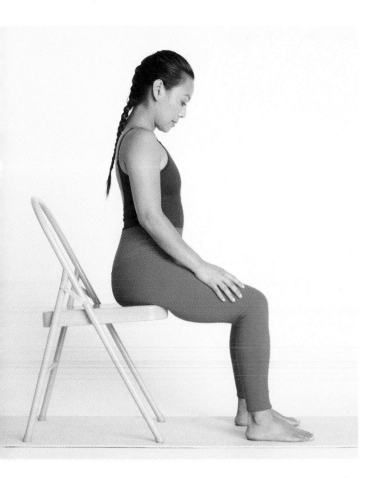

FIGURE 2.8

pose well, and to practice it with knowledge, we need to understand the normal range of motion in the cervical spine.

Every moveable joint in the body has a normal range of motion. This range is limited by the shape of the joint and by the soft tissue, like ligaments, tendons, and the joint capsule. These structures can be tight or loose or can be injured or diseased in some way. But generally, there is an accepted and measurable number that reflects the normal range of motion for each joint.

The normal range of motion of flexion for the neck (forward bending) is about 55°. To feel this amount of flexion, sit at the front of a chair with your feet flat on the floor and all your normal curves intact. Make sure your lumbar curve is not rounded, i.e., you are not slumping, but instead are sitting with your weight slightly in front of your sitting bones. Make sure your head is directly over your body.

Now flex your neck, easily letting your chin drop toward your chest. Do not recruit any movement from the upper thoracic spine; do not disturb the curves or round the back. Isolate this movement entirely to the neck. You will find that the chin does not reach the chest. That true neck flexion is *not* 90°, or anywhere close to that, which many people are surprised to learn.

Lift your head so the neck is in neutral again. Now try to gently move your chin all the way into your chest without forcing this movement or creating any discomfort or pain. You will only be able to do this if you flex or round your upper back as well. When you do this, notice that your entire spine now collapses a bit, and that your shoulders are rounding forward.

Is this the posture you want to have in Shoulder Stand, with almost all the weight of your body resting on your lower cervical vertebrae, especially on the C7 and T1 area? While sitting or standing, gently place your fingers on the base of your neck at the back and feel how the lower cervical and upper thoracic vertebrae are prominent. This is the location where the weight of your body is falling if Shoulder Stand is practiced without support. Notice this in figure 2.9.

There is a way to avoid this situation. Practicing Shoulder Stand with blanket support under the shoulders can solve the problem.

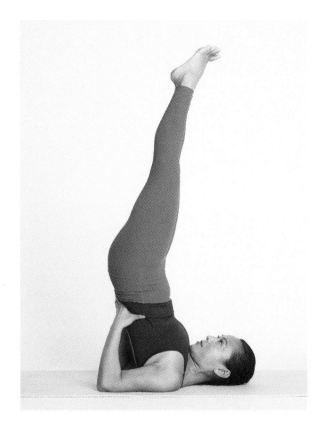

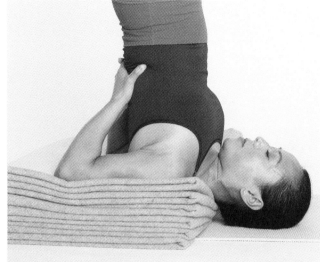

FIGURE 2.9

FIGURE 2.10

Elevating the shoulders creates three advantages in the pose. First, the normal range of motion is preserved. Note in figure 2.10 that the model's neck is at approximately 55° of flexion. In this position, the back of the neck feels soft to the touch, and some students can slightly lift the neck off the floor if their feet are on the wall taking most of the weight off the neck in the pose. There is "play" in the tissues of the cervical spine. The joints and soft tissues are not stretched to the end of their range.

Second, with blankets as support there is little, if any, weight on the neck itself. The weight is being borne by the shoulders. And isn't the name of the pose "Shoulder Stand"? When the weight is borne by the shoulders, it is distributed across the shoulders where there is a wider base of support with larger muscles to protect the area.

Third, the upper thoracic curve and vertebrae are not as likely to be compromised when we practice with blankets. The chest is not collapsing, breathing is easier, and the practitioner is more at ease. In the Yoga Sutras of Patanjali, Pada 2, verse 46, the author defines asana as: "abiding in ease is asana." Thus according to Patanjali, there are two qualities an asana must have: stillness and ease.

When both the cervical and the thoracic spine are at ease and not pushed past their normal range of motion or asked to bear weight in a precarious way, and when the breath is free, one is more likely to be "still and at ease."

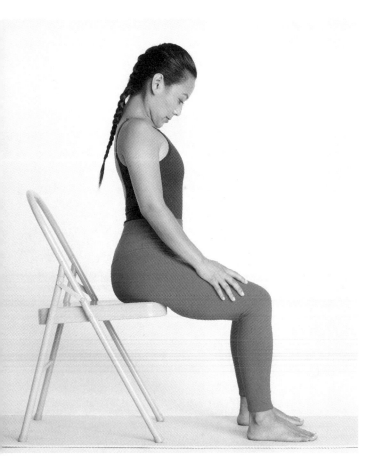

FIGURE 2.11

Please study the model in figure 2.10. Notice how the chest and neck are very different in shape from figure 2.9. Practicing with blankets is prophylactic: it minimizes the chances of strain and injury, and it maximizes the chances of ease and presence in the pose.

In the "Attentive Practice" section, we will learn to practice Shoulder Stand with blankets and at the wall in a safe and comfortable manner. But first a word about *jalandhara bandha*.

Jalandhara is a word that basically means "net"; a bandha is a lock. When one practices a bandha, it is for the purpose of holding or directing energy in the body. Jalandhara is one of the three main bandha, the other two being *uddihyana* bandha (abdominal lock) and the aforementioned mula bandha.

Often jalandhara bandha is taught in Shoulder Stand explicitly by telling students to press the chin to the chest. I have found a different way of practicing and teaching jalandhara bandha.

Please sit again with all your spinal curves intact and with the head directly over the body. Now with care and attention, gently bring the chin to the chest. You will notice that now your cervical and thoracic spines both round, and the throat will feel tight and closed. This is not the bandha, because a bandha is about directing energy and is not just a purely physical action. You will notice that if you try to talk in this position, your voice will be muffled and strained.

Lift your head to the beginning position again. This time just drop the head so your neck is resting in no more than 55° of flexion. Now lift your breastbone with a slight backbend of your mid-back.

Now you are bringing the chest to the chin instead of the chin to the chest, and the sensation and awareness is completely different. If you attempt to speak with the head and neck in this position, the voice will be lightly affected, but there is no sense of strain or effort. And the high part of the sternum near the chin will feel broad, the skin there will seem to be moving toward the sides of your body, while the mind is drawn into quietness. This is jalandhara bandha. (Note figure 2.10 again.)

My suggestion is that during Shoulder Stand, the best way to create a comfortable bandha is to bring the chest to the chin, which is much more easily created by placing blankets under the shoulders and allowing the neck to be free and at 55° of flexion, and the chest to be open and moving toward the chin.

Attentive Practice

Remember, the cervical spine is both the most mobile and most delicate of all the regions of the vertebral column. Approach the practices suggested below with respect for your neck and with curiosity for how intelligently it moves to bear the weight of the head.

CAUTIONS

If you feel any pain or discomfort when trying these neck movements, consider a consultation with your health-care provider before practicing them. Avoid these neck movements if you have radiating pain in your neck, shoulder, or arm, or if you have a neck injury; for example, if you are recovering from whiplash.

There are ways to stretch your neck area pleasantly without pain and without doing neck rolls. The main principle here is to do one movement in one direction at a time, and only move as far as is pain free for you.

In other words, the stretches given below will only be unidirectional. Be sure to move slowly and pay attention to the *process* of practicing the movement, not just to how far you can go. Remember to pay attention to how the movement feels and only move slowly and with awareness.

Please note that besides these general cautions, there are special cautions offered below for Shoulder Stand. Please adhere to these cautions carefully.

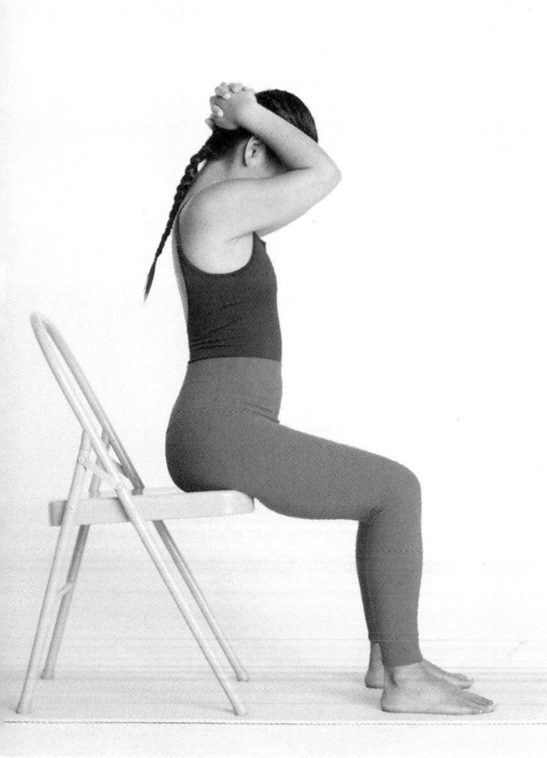

Neck Stretch 1

FLEXION

Sit on your mat or the front half of the seat of a chair with your feet flat on the floor. Make sure that your spinal column is long, and all its natural curves are intact. Bring your chin exactly parallel to the floor.

Inhale, and with an exhalation, drop your chin so your face is exactly parallel to the floor. At the end of your range, take a breath.

Then interlock your fingers, and place your hands on the back of your head, letting your elbows drop as well.

Gradually let the weight of your hands and forearms increase the stretch slightly; remember to use your exhalation when you do this. This is a passive stretch. Do not pull your head down; just let gravity and the weight of the arms do the work. After a couple of breaths, let go of your hands and arms, and raise your head up. Notice the release in the muscles of the back of your neck. Under no circumstances force the flexion of the neck. Remember to be gentle with yourself at all times.

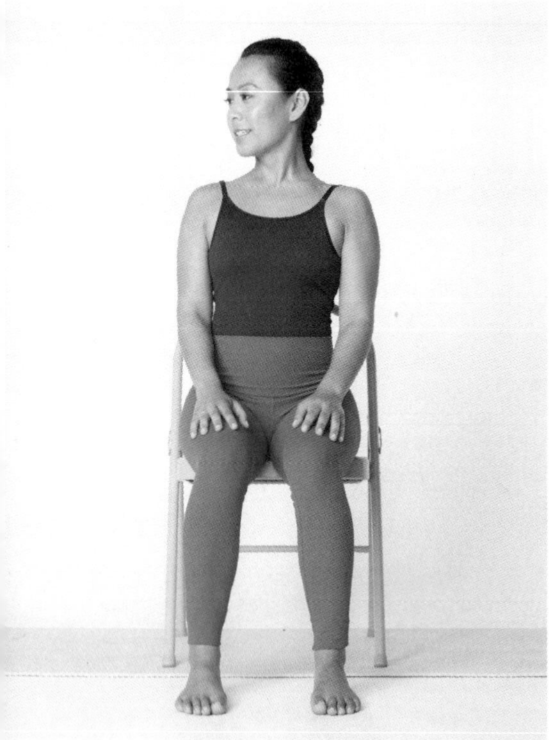

FIGURE 2.12

Neck Stretch 2

ROTATION

Sit on your yoga mat or the front half of the seat of a chair with your feet flat on the floor. Make sure that your spinal column is long, and all its natural curves are intact. Bring your chin exactly parallel to the floor.

Inhale, and with an exhalation, slowly turn to your right until you feel a slight "block" to the movement. Stay there and take one full breath. Then try to rotate a little farther on the next exhalation and hold this new position for a breath. Be careful not to force your neck. Do not let the chin lift; keep it absolutely parallel to the floor. Repeat on the left side.

FIGURE 2.13

Neck Stretch 3

SIDE BENDING

Sit on your yoga mat or the front half of the seat of a chair with your feet flat on the floor. Make sure that your spinal column is long, and all its natural curves are intact. Bring your chin exactly parallel to the floor.

Inhale, and as you exhale, bend your right ear toward your right shoulder while letting your chin roll slowly down with the bend.

You will be looking down toward the floor a bit as you side bend. Take at least two breaths and come up with an exhalation. Be sure you are *not keeping your face looking forward, but are turning it downward.* Repeat the stretch to the left.

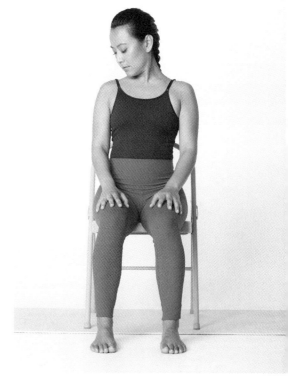

FIGURE 2.14

Neck Stretch 4

VISUALIZATION

Sit on your yoga mat or the front half of the seat of a chair with your feet flat on the floor. Make sure that your spinal column is long, and all its natural curves are intact. Bring your chin exactly parallel to the floor.

Begin by rotating your head to the right as explained above. When you have gone as far as is comfortable, use your eyes to mark a place on the wall or on a piece of furniture so you can remember how far you turned.

Now come back to the starting position with your chin parallel to the floor. Keep your head in this position and close your eyes. This time you are not going to actually move your head and neck at all, but are only going *to think about moving.* Begin to count slowly from one to twenty. On each count, imagine your head rotating to the right, while it actually is remaining still.

When you are done, and your head and neck are in the starting position, open your eyes. Now actually physically rotate your head to the right. You will be surprised how much farther you can rotate after visualizing it twenty times. Repeat to the left.

Supported Shoulder Stand Pose

SALAMBA SARVANGASANA

Shoulder Stand is one of the most classic and delicious poses in all of asana practice. Be meticulous with your setup, and you will likely come to deeply enjoy the physical and mental effects of this pose.

SPECIAL CAUTIONS FOR SHOULDER STAND POSE

Avoid this asana if you have radiating pain in your neck, shoulder, or arm, or if you have a neck injury; for example, if you are recovering from whiplash. If at all possible, please learn this pose with a qualified yoga teacher present. Do not practice this pose if you have or are recovering from a throat or ear infection, are menstruating or pregnant, or have gastric reflux, glaucoma, retinal tears, or high blood pressure. And if you have any concerns at all about turning upside down, consult your health professional before practicing this pose. This pose is intended for healthy experienced yoga students.

ADDITIONAL PROPS NEEDED FOR SHOULDER STAND

Learning to practice Shoulder Stand with blankets will take some time, and you will need the following props:

- Nonslip yoga mat
- Smooth empty wall

- At least five, and possibly more, firm yoga blankets. The number of blankets needed for your pose is not completely predictable due to the variation in the thickness of blankets. Some students use anywhere from six to nine blankets. I prefer firm cotton Mexican yoga blankets. Wool yoga blankets will work, too. If you are allergic to wool, you can still use wool blankets by simply placing a cotton blanket on top of the stack. The key is that the blankets you use should not be plush, but quite firm.

Begin by placing your yoga mat near a plain wall. Fold your blankets into the shape shown in figure 2.15 and place them near the wall. Make sure that your blankets are exactly stacked one on top of another so that their edges are exactly in line. It may take a time or two to get the right blanket height and the right distance from the wall for your particular body proportions.

Now look below at the photos of the model rolling onto the blankets so as to be positioned near the wall for the pose. The first time or two you try this, it is likely that you will have to come down and adjust your proximity to the

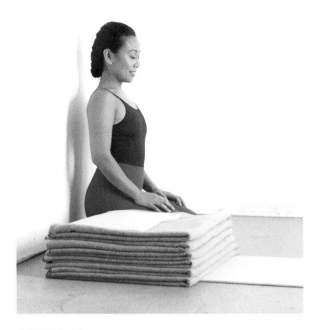

FIGURE 2.15

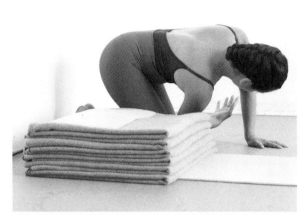

FIGURE 2.16

wall by moving the blankets either closer or far-ther from the wall. Be patient. You will learn the correct distance for you quite quickly.

Once you are settled on your blankets, make sure the tops of your shoulders are about three to four inches from the edge of the blankets. This will vary by individual, but the reason some space is needed is that you are going to roll slowly onto the top of your shoulders, and you still want to be on the blankets when you do so.

Place your feet on the wall, about ten to twelve inches apart. Inhale and gradually begin to curl up. This is an important instruction. Many times, students push so much with their legs that they push themselves toward the center of the room and thus off the mat. Be careful to avoid this. Keep the shoulders still and firmly held on the blankets as you curl up.

Use your abdominal muscles and curl slowly instead of pushing with your legs, which would end up moving you away from the wall. This is not what you want to do. You want all the motion to be an upward one of your legs, pelvis, and chest.

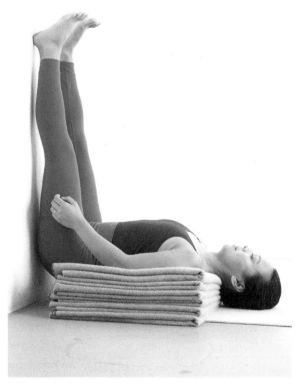

FIGURE 2.17

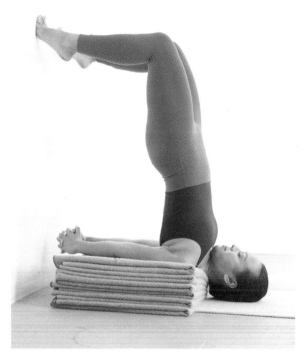

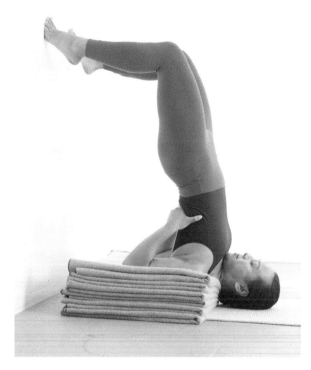

FIGURE 2.18   FIGURE 2.19

Interlock your hands behind your back, straighten your elbows, and push downward with your arms as you lift.

Turn your upper arms out, in external rotation. You may want to tuck your outer upper arms under you a bit, one by one, by rocking gently side to side as you do so.

When you are all the way up on the top of your shoulders, take a breath or two. Slowly place your hands on your back so that your thumbs are pointing around toward the front of your body and your hands are parallel with the ribs. The space between the thumbs and your index finger is pressing into your rib cage.

Imagine that the ribs are a "ladder," and that your hands are climbing down the ladder as far as they can go. Press downward strongly with your upper arms while you lift firmly with your hands. Remember to breathe slowly.

Have your teacher tell you if your lower legs are horizontal to the wall and your knees are bent at a 90° angle. Your sternum should be vertical and your throat at ease. It is crucial that your head is lower than your shoulders and that your neck is at a 55° angle and feels completely free.

Stay here for five breaths. Each time you try this pose at the wall, stay in the pose for a few more breaths. After you have practiced with your feet on the wall enough times that it feels familiar and comfortable, then you are ready to do the pose with your feet away from the wall. Ask your teacher to stand by you and help you to take first one leg and then the other away from the wall. This is the way you will come back to the wall, one foot at a time before you roll out.

Do not move your legs unless you are firmly holding your back with your hands, whether you are going up or coming down. Be sure to lift through the balls of the feet, internally rotate your thighs, and keep the legs straight. Always turn your eyes downward toward your heart and keep your focus inward while you are in the pose. The sternum is always lifting up in Shoulder Stand, never sinking. If you cannot do this with your legs away from the wall, try adding another blanket.

You can gradually work up to staying for five minutes in Supported Shoulder Stand if you are in good health and have no neck conditions. Every once in a while, have an experienced teacher give you some feedback on your alignment in the pose.

When you're are ready to come down, release your hands, open your arms to the side a bit, pressing them down to help control the speed of descent, and roll down. Once down on the blankets, move gently off your mat toward the center of the room until your shoulders are on the floor.

Stay there with your knees bent and your feet on the floor for several breaths. Notice the sense of calmness in your mind and openness in your chest. When you are ready, roll to the side and sit up slowly. Many students like to practice Deep Relaxation Pose after Shoulder Stand, or perhaps a Supported Forward Bend.

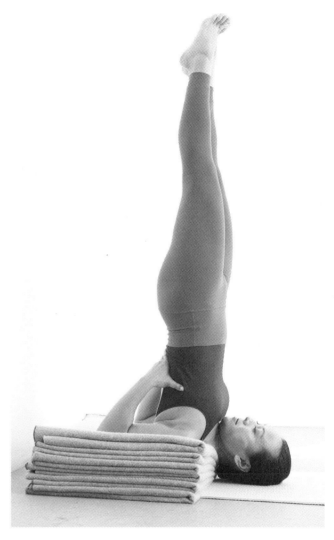

FIGURE 2.20

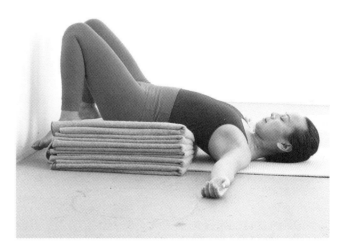

FIGURE 2.21

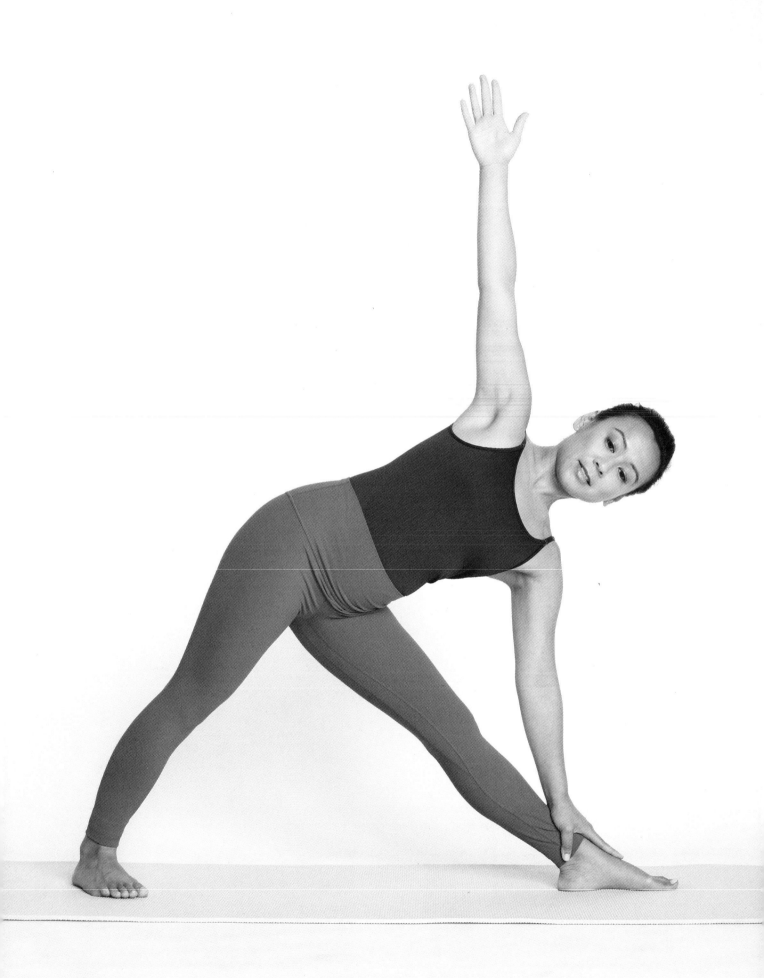

3

Free Your Pelvis and Spine, Part 1

STANDING POSES AND BACKBENDS

The pelvis is the pot out of which the spine grows.

D URING PHYSICAL THERAPY SCHOOL, my classmates and I spent time observing the specifics of how each other walked as a way of training our eyes to see how muscles and joints work together to create the symphony of movement. As our proficiency grew, we could clearly see who had tight calf muscles, whose sacroiliac joint was not moving symmetrically, and whose pelvis was too rigidly held, just by doing this visual gait analysis. We thought it was a fun game.

On my first trip to India to study yoga a few years later, I was struck by the stark differences between my culture and India's. The most noteworthy of these differences for me was revealed during my frequent habit of people watching. My specific fascination was watching people simply walk down the street, especially the women. Many of them carried baskets or pots on their head, and their effortlessly elegant posture and fluid movement was mesmerizing.

What was so striking to me in my informal cross-cultural gait analysis was how easily these Indian women initiated walking from their pelvis, not their legs. The pelvis was not only the origin of their walking, but also the root of their spine as it flowed upward so that their head was lightly and exactly held over their body. It looked like they were dancing rather than walking.

When I returned home to the United States after five weeks in India, I noticed with fresh eyes how most people walked. It was not from the pelvis, it was from the legs only, and it often looked like walking was laborious. It did not have the natural grace I saw demonstrated by many of the people I had observed in India.

I became even more fascinated with the importance of the pelvis in walking, standing, sitting, and in virtually all movements we make in the course of the day. Taking this awareness to my yoga mat transformed my asana practice. I learned a simple fact: the pelvis is the key to every asana, especially the position of the vertebral column. Trying to keep the movements of the column and pelvis separate is a yoga myth.

Why You Need to Know This

The key to the walking I saw in India was clearly the pelvis. The pelvis is not only at the center of our body, not only the site of many important physiological functions, not only the cradle of new life, but is also the crossroads of the upper body and lower body. The pelvis is the true site where our locomotion begins.

The position of your pelvis at any given moment creates and affects the position of your vertebral column, and especially of the neck and the head. Try this. Whatever position you are sitting in right now as you read this book, move your pelvis in any direction one inch. Notice how your spinal column adjusts immediately. That is why pelvic position is so important in a meditation posture, but its position is of primary importance in standing and walking as well.

Additionally, the position of your pelvis also dictates the position of your legs, knees, and feet. In fluid walking, the pelvis moves, and the legs and spine follow. I often tell my students to think of walking from the pelvis first and letting everything else follow. I say this because almost all of our movements, both in our daily lives and on our yoga mat, originate from the pelvis.

In this chapter, we will focus on the position of the pelvis in standing poses and backbends in yoga asana. Learning to move from the pelvis in both these types of poses is healthier for your vertebral column and makes standing poses and backbends easier and more pleasant. But first we need to review a little anatomy.

Your Structure

The pelvis is made of three bones strongly connected and working together as one bony ring. These three bones are the ilium, the ischium, and the pubic bone. Both the ischium and the pubic bone have two rami, or arms.

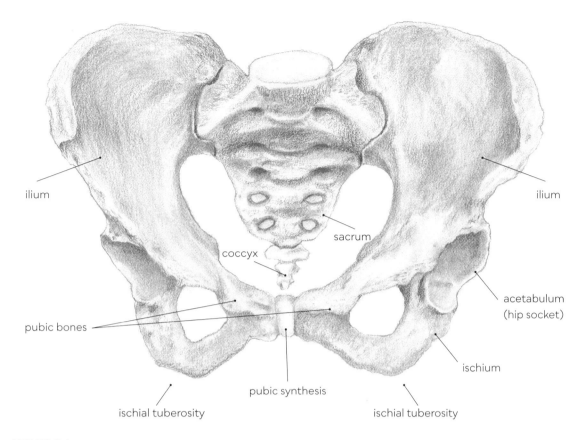

ilium

ilium

sacrum

coccyx

acetabulum
(hip socket)

pubic bones

ischium

ischial tuberosity

pubic synthesis

ischial tuberosity

FIGURE 3.1

You can feel your ilium along both sides of your body below your waist. It is a broad curving bone and the largest of the three pelvic bones. The pubic bone connects to the other two bones from the lowest part of your abdomen. The two rami are joined together at the pubic symphysis and held strongly together by ligaments and cartilage. The ischium is the third bone and often referred to as the "sitting bones." You have felt your sitting bones if you have gone horseback riding when you are not used to it. The very tip of the ischium is where three of the four hamstrings attach.

The word *pelvis* means "basin," and the pelvis functions, in part, as a basin that holds and protects your deep abdominal organs. The back of this basin is formed in part by the sacrum, the final curved bone of the spinal column. This is where the column transfers weight into the pelvis and down through the lower extremities. The pelvis and the column work together in all daily activities and yoga poses.

In addition to this symbiotic relationship between the pelvis and the sacrum, the pelvis joins below with the top of the femur (thighbone) bone to form the hip joint. All three bones of the pelvis join together to form the acetabulum, the concave receiving, or socket, part of the hip joint. The ilium makes up two-thirds of the acetabulum, and the pubic bone and ischium bones make up one-third each.

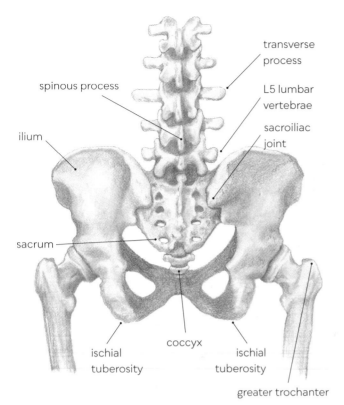

transverse process

L5 lumbar vertebrae

sacroiliac joint

spinous process

ilium

sacrum

ischial tuberosity

coccyx

ischial tuberosity

greater trochanter

FIGURE 3.2

The pelvis translates the movements of the hip joint to the spine, trunk, upper extremities, and head. The opposite is also true: the weight and movements of the spinal column, and of structures above it, are translated directly through the pelvis into the thighs, legs, and feet.

Your Anatomy in Action

One of the most common types of poses we learn when we begin asana practice is the broad category of poses termed "standing poses." This makes intuitive and logical sense. Human beings, unlike almost all other mammals, stand and walk on only two legs. Focusing on the yoga poses that are most like our daily lives, poses that stretch and strengthen the muscles of the legs, hips, and lower trunk, challenge balance and free the spinal column, and as such, are worth time and focus.

I like to say, "If you can walk, you can do standing poses." It may be, however, that some students, or many of us at different times in our life, may need to use a wall, chair, or yoga block in our standing-pose practice. Even when we need a little extra help, the standing poses are the basis of our practice, and rightfully so.

Figure 3.3 shows one of the most basic standing poses: Standing Forward Bend (Uttanasana). This pose looks simple but requires some real understanding of the relationship of the lower extremities, the hip joint, and the spinal column as they work together to allow us to bend forward.

Just like the vertebral column is a kinetic chain that moves as a whole, so too is the lower extremity. Each part affects the other parts. To feel this in your body in Standing Forward Bend, unroll your mat and step on. You may want a block or even two to support your hands. Place your feet about ten to fourteen inches apart and turn your feet out so that your toes are pointing away from each other.

Keeping your knees straight, try to bend forward. You will feel blocked. Come up, and try the pose again, but this time with your toes turning inward, heels turning slightly out. Now the pose has become so much easier. Here's

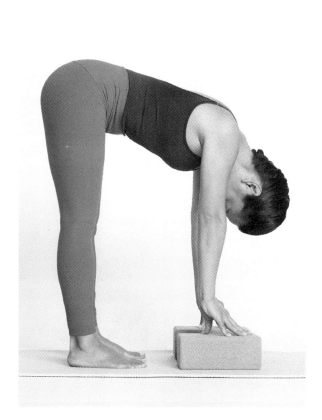

FIGURE 3.3

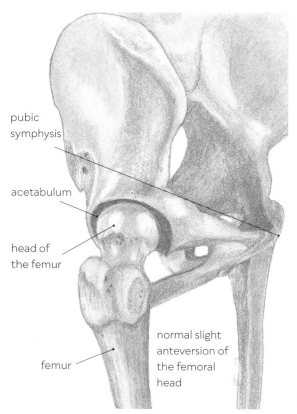

pubic
symphysis

acetabulum

head of
the femur

femur

normal slight
anteversion of
the femoral
head

FIGURE 3.4

why: Most yoga students do not know that the acetabulum points slightly forward, not laterally, toward the side of the body. The actual forward angle of the hip joint is about 15° and is called anteversion. This means that the socket of your hip joint points slightly forward as does the greater trochanter. This slight anteversion angle is normal and does vary some from person to person. The shape and depth of the hip joint can also vary a fair amount across populations and usually by gender as well.

In standing, in order for the feet to turn out, the femurs must be externally rotated. Externally rotating your thighs is the only way you can turn your feet out. There is no other way to do it. With an externally rotated femoral head in the hip joint, it is more difficult for the acetabulum to move forward and down over the tops of the femurs to create flexion in the hip joint.

I suggest that when practicing Standing Forward Bend, and all seated forward bends, you always internally rotate the femurs to facilitate flexion. You can experiment in other forward-bending poses like Seated Forward Bend (Paschimottanasana). Notice how internal rotation of the femurs affects your ability to bend forward. It's not just your hamstrings that limit this movement.

There is, however, much more going on in the body in this asana, besides what is happening in the hip joints, that allows us to create the final pose. Not only do the hip joints need to move easily over the femoral heads, but the entire pelvis also needs to tip forward. The position of the feet, turning inward or outward, is created by the rotation of the femurs, internally or externally, and this rotation also directly affects the position of the pelvis.

With the feet turned out and the thighs externally rotated, the action in the hip joint is incomplete and blocked, and therefore the pelvis does not move fully forward and down. The result is that now the thoracic and lumbar spines are flexed (rounded) at the exact angle that is the most stressful for the muscles and intervertebral discs in those areas. The internal rotation of the femurs and inward turn of the toes facilitates hip flexion that allows the pelvis to move, which frees the spinal column. We need to learn to practice and to teach others how to bend forward from the hips and pelvis and not the spinal column.

Try this experiment. Take your yoga mat to a section of clear wall and place the short end of the mat against the wall. You may also want to take a yoga block or two to support your hands and arms when you bend forward.

Now place your tailbone against the wall with your feet about twelve to fourteen inches from the wall and ten to fourteen inches apart from each other, and toes turning inward slightly. Lean back so that you know exactly where your tailbone is on the wall. Place your hands close to your side thighs, drop your chin, and while you exhale, bend forward by focusing on pressing and lifting your tailbone on the wall, as you drag it upward. Feel the pressure of the tailbone on the wall the whole time you are moving. Keep your knees straight.

Stop immediately when your tailbone is no longer moving upward. If your back pelvis and sacrum are not well below a 90° angle, this means your lumbar spine and discs are now experiencing a tremendous shearing force of gravity, especially at the lower lumbar area. This is not a healthy forward bend, even if you succeed in touching the floor. The movement of forward bending needs to come from the pelvis, not the lower back.

In figure 3.5 B, the model is demonstrating how the Standing Forward Bend is done when a student who has looser hamstrings bends forward. Because there is more looseness in the back thigh muscles, the pelvis is able to tip forward easier, thus reducing strain on the lower back structures.

If the rounding shown in figure 3.5 is happening when you practice the pose, please practice the following alternative pose instead. Face the wall with your feet the same distance apart as before, and your thighs rotated inward, heels slightly rotated outward. Keep your knees straight and make sure that your pelvis is directly over your feet in the pose. Place your hands on the wall

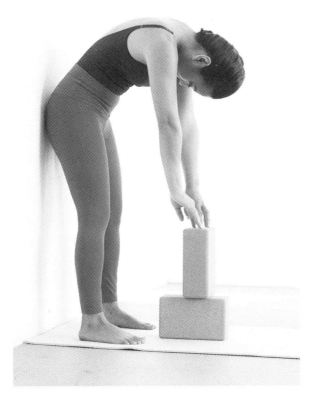

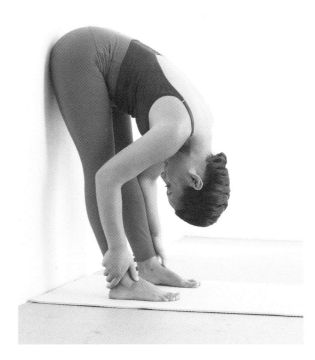

FIGURE 3.5

FIGURE 3.5B

at shoulder height and slightly wider than your shoulders. Point your fingers upward and open them apart slightly. Press your thumb and index finger slightly more into the wall than the rest of the palm. Now bend forward by walking backward slowly, until you come to a place where you feel a pleasant stretch in the middle of your back thighs.

Your trunk might be at a 90° angle to the floor, but this is not the most important thing. The most important thing to remain safe and happy in this pose is for the pelvis to be rotating forward so the sacrum is parallel to the floor. This variation will create a healthy stretch for the hamstrings if they are tight. Hold for five breaths, then with an inhalation, walk your body toward the wall to come up. Always remember to listen to your body and never force forward bends by bending your knees or rounding the lumbar and thoracic spines against gravity.

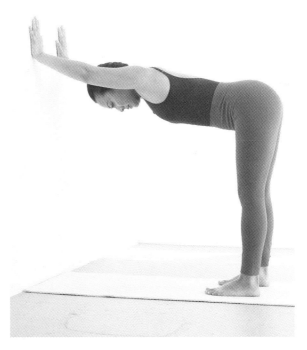

FIGURE 3.6

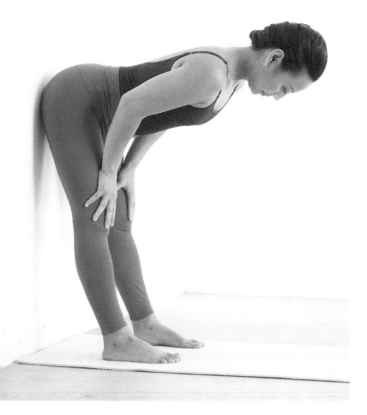

FIGURE 3.7

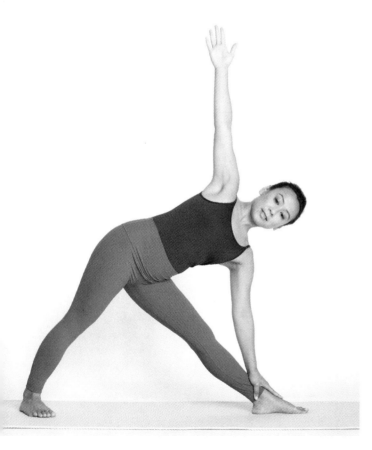

FIGURE 3.8

If your back is well below the horizontal in Standing Forward Bend with your pelvis at the wall (like the model in figure 3.5 B), then let your arms come down, fingers on the floor or on the block, keep your chin dropped, and breathe five to ten breaths before coming up, engaging your hamstrings. Keep your arms at your side as you come up. Be absolutely meticulous to maintain your normal curves as you come up.

Another common pose that can help us to understand the natural movement of the hip joints, pelvis, and vertebral column is Triangle Pose (Trikonasana).

Just about everyone who has studied modern asana practice in the West has been taught Triangle Pose. While I do teach this pose to beginners, I have found that it is more subtle and complicated, anatomically and kinesiologically, than is commonly known.

One of the yoga myths that I encounter almost everywhere in the world I teach is that Triangle Pose is to be practiced as if we are moving "between two panes of glass." This is the exact phrase students tell me, no matter the state, country, or continent where the class is taking place. I disagree with this image and this instruction, and do not like the pose this image creates, and here's why.

The pose is meant to be a pose primarily from the movement of the hip joints, not just the vertebral column, as are all standing poses. When Triangle Pose is practiced as suggested above, the student is holding her pelvis still and trying to side bend. This allows very little movement from the hip joints.

The premise behind moving in a flat plane like between two panes of glass does not take into account that the hip joints are rounded surfaces. Not only is the acetabulum a rounded concave surface, but the heads of the femurs are round as well. Movement in this joint occurs in arcs, not straight lines.

Neither does this "two planes of glass" instruction take into account the fact that the pelvis is basically a bony ring. The three bones of the pelvis, as explained above, are joined in the front of the body at the pubic symphysis and on the posterior side through the sacroiliac joints. There is slight movement (measured in millimeters) at both places when we walk and move from sitting to standing and standing to sitting, and especially at the pubic symphysis when we squat. There is much greater mobility at the sacroiliac joints and the pubic joint during pregnancy, birth, and the nursing period.

Basically, sacroiliac joints are joints of stability *not* mobility. In fact, sacroiliac pain is usually caused by too much laxity around the joint, probably due to overstretching and/or injuring the supporting ligaments in the area. Too much laxity allows the joint to move around too much. When this happens, the joint surfaces cannot offer much stability because they are not congruent, that is lightly touching as much as is possible within the limits of the movement needed. Then what is left is for the soft tissue around the joint, like ligaments, to compensate by trying to hold the joint together. This can cause the soft tissue to become chronically stressed and irritated, leading to pain and eventual joint dysfunction in the long term.

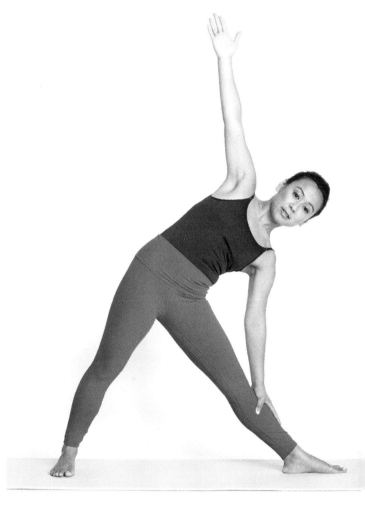

FIGURE 3.9

We cannot move our right pelvis to the right and our left pelvis to the left at the same time in Triangle Pose, like we were opening a book. That is simply not how the body works. It would be somewhat like trying to move the right side of a bowl to the right and simultaneously the left side of the bowl to the left. The bowl would break.

Our pelvis doesn't break, but we can be injured when the back hip is held "back" while coming into the pose as well as trying to turn the front pelvis in the opposite direction. When we attempt to do this unnatural movement, some other part of the body has to compensate; it is usually the ligaments of the sacroiliac joints, the lumbar spine, and/or the hip joint itself that take the brunt. In the "Attentive Practice" section below, another approach to moving the pelvis in Triangle Pose will be taught.

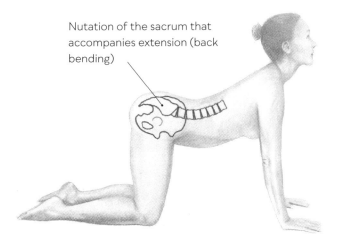

Nutation of the sacrum that accompanies extension (back bending)

FIGURE 3.10

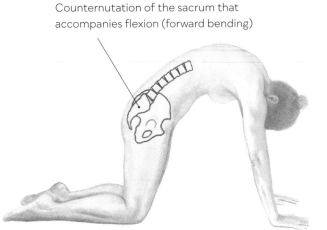

Counternutation of the sacrum that accompanies flexion (forward bending)

FIGURE 3.11

The pelvis and hip joints play a major part in backbending poses as well. The position of the pelvis in backbends can change the way the lumbosacral spine moves and thus affect the rest of the column, shoulder joints, and neck.

A very common instruction in yoga asana is to "tuck the tailbone" in backbends to "protect the back." Obviously thinking of tucking the tailbone changes the position of the pelvis, and thus the vertebral column. When we change the position of the pelvis, we directly affect the function of the back.

You may enjoy rereading the first part of chapter 1 at this point, especially the story relayed there. Remember that the student at the center of the story found that bringing her pelvis into a neutral position in standing created the normal position of the entire vertebral column and thus more stability in the pose.

The pelvis and vertebral column work harmoniously together like this in backbends as well. But because we can more easily see, feel, and understand pelvic movements, we will focus on the pelvis in backbends here.

When the tailbone is allowed to move upward, toward the ceiling, the top sacrum (S1 vertebral segment) moves down toward the floor. This is a movement called nutation, from the Latin *nutare*, which means "to nod." The top of the sacrum is nodding forward toward the front of the body. This is the natural movement of the sacrum; it passively follows the extension or backbending of the lumbar spine.

These two movements always go together in your body unless you purposively override them. If you sit in a chair and press your pubic bone down to the front seat of the chair, your lumbar spine backbends, and your top sacrum follows it by nodding forward. If you round your back in flexion so your pelvis now tips backward and your belly sinks in, this is called counternutation, or tucking the tailbone. Counternutation always accompanies flexion. It is a natural and healthy movement for the lower back in flexion, not extension.

The sacrum nutates and counternutates as it follows the movements of the lumbar spine and pelvis in all positions of the body: vertical, horizontal, or somewhere in between. If you pay attention during your yoga asana practice, as well as in the movements you make in daily life, you will begin to notice this passive movement more and more.

Nutation follows lumbar extension, and counternutation follows flexion. There are no muscles that create these movements, and nutation and counternutation are not created separately from lumbar extension and flexion unless you interfere from your conscious mind. These movements are therefore what we call "passive joint movements." The sacrum passively follows the lumbar unless you override that movement.

Remember, your body is smarter than you are. To move without pain or injury, and with the natural laws of the body in backbends, allow the sacrum to nutate. Your lumbar and sacroiliac joints will thank you.

MAIN POINTS TO REMEMBER FROM THIS CHAPTER

→ The position of your pelvis at any given moment creates and affects the position of your vertebral column and vice versa.

→ The pelvis is a bony ring and moves as a whole piece: when one side moves, the other side always does too.

→ Let your sacrum and lumbar spine move in their natural rhythm; do not tuck during backbends.

Attentive Practice

Try to think of all standing movements, whether they are in your asana practice or in the movements of daily life, as originating from the pelvis and that the spinal column always follows the pelvis.

CAUTIONS

If you feel any pain with these poses, in your knees, ankle, or back especially, come out and seek out a trained teacher before you continue. Remember, there is no healthy pain in a joint. You may want to consider a consultation with your health-care provider before continuing.

PROPS NEEDED

- Nonslip yoga mat
- Two yoga blocks
- Folded yoga blanket

Extended Triangle Pose
UTTHITA TRIKONASANA

Roll out your yoga mat and step on. Then take a breath or two.

Now separate your feet as demonstrated in figure 3.12. Turn your right toes toward you so that they point inward. Now turn your left foot out a little more than 90° so your toes slightly point toward the wall behind you.

If you are using blocks, place your block on the outside of your left foot; this is a good idea if you are a beginning student. If you are using two blocks, it is more stable if you place the bottom block in the low position. The second block can be either in the medium or tall positions.

When you turn your left leg out, note that it is the entire leg that is turning out from your left hip joint to turn the whole thigh. The knee turns as well, as does the tibia. Make sure that as much as possible your left kneecap is facing toward the back wall and not forward over your big toe. Your left kneecap is in alignment exactly with your left foot below it.

When you start this pose with the feet and legs aligned as described above, your pelvis *must* be turning with you. Your left pelvis is turning to the left completely, and your right pelvis is coming passively with you. Do not force the right pelvis to turn. You will likely overdo it. Rather, just *allow* the natural intelligence of the pelvis to assert itself, and your pelvis will turn just the right amount. Your trunk will be slightly turned to the left as well.

In this position you are not holding your left pelvis back, you are not thinking of moving between two panes of glass, and you are not trying to do the impossible with your pelvis. You are simply allowing the healthy and natural movement of the acetabula over the femoral heads as was meant to happen when you go into the pose.

I once had an experienced student get tears in her eyes in class and tell me that when she allowed her pelvis to move naturally in Triangle Pose as was suggested, and did not collapse it forward, it was the first time in ten years that she did not have pain in her front hip joint in the pose. We always suffer when we go against our body's natural intelligence. Your hip joint is smarter than you.

Now raise your arms out to your sides so that they are parallel to the floor and stretch them away from you. Begin this stretch at the scapula. Keeping your legs absolutely straight, inhale, and coordinating breath and movement, exhale and gradually stretch mostly out away from you. To a lesser degree stretch down. Allow your right pelvis to swing back toward your right leg, and place your left hand on your ankle or on the block.

If you are using a block, use your fingertips to press into the block instead of your palm. The use of the fingertips will remind you that the emphasis of the action is on moving the energy of the right arm *upward,* not on hanging down on the left arm or collapsing the shoulders to touch the floor or the block.

It is perfectly fine, and many times more effective and pleasant, not to strive to go down too far. Make sure that you have built up enough height with the block so that you can stay in the pose for several breaths and enjoy yourself. If not, come up and change your block.

In the pose remember to look straight ahead, not to turn your head up or down, and to breathe naturally. Stretch out in all directions like a star: press the back foot down, especially the front of your left heel at the beginning of your arch, move the arms apart from one another as well as your shoulder blades, and let the left side of your trunk drop down. Move your shoulder blades away from your ears.

Your right pelvis is now very slightly dropping forward in the pose. Look again at the model's back hip position in figure 3.13. When you are in this position, your navel is slightly facing downward. Move your very top right thigh backward slightly into your body to feel the grounding energy, especially equally and evenly at the outer and inner back foot. Do not distort your ankle.

Now inhale, and with an exhalation, keep the frame of your trunk still. This means that you are keeping your shoulder girdle and pelvis still while you turn the soft belly, heart, and lungs to your left, opening them upward.

Another image of this is to think of the bones remaining still, and the soft body swirling from your back and side waist forward and around toward the heavens to open your front body. Your chest follows this energetic movement of the belly as well. This is the true opening of the pose. Come up while you inhale and then repeat on the opposite side.

When you turn your soft body with your pelvis in this position, you will not strain or injure your lumbosacral spine. However, you will likely begin to love this pose and want to practice it more.

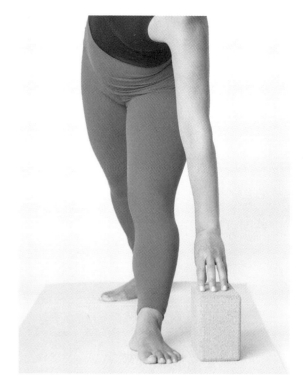

FIGURE 3.12

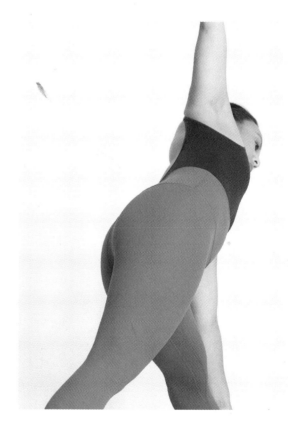

FIGURE 3.13

Extended Side Angle Pose

UTTHITA PARSVAKONASANA

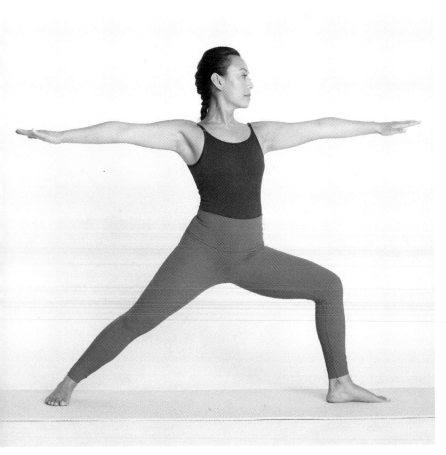

FIGURE 3.14

Step onto your mat and place your feet wider apart than for Triangle Pose, approximately three-and-a-half feet, or very slightly more. Place a block on the outside of your right foot at the height you think you might need. Turn your left foot out a little more than 90° and your right foot in about halfway. Keep the weight on the outside of your back foot and mostly on the back part of the front foot; the ball of your left foot can bear some weight, but the toes are resting on the floor relatively lightly. Raise your arms to the side.

Begin by inhaling, and as you exhale, bend your left knee over you left little toe; bring your thigh down to as close to parallel to the floor as you can without strain.

Pause here, and without moving the position of the legs, exhale as you stretch out with your left arm to place your fingers for support on your block.

Your fingers should be firm; do not rest on your palm. Imagine you are lifting up a bit off the block. Stretch your right arm in a diagonal line past your head. Let your shoulder blade move out with the arm. Do not hold it back; set it free.

Tuck your chin and turn your head to look straight ahead. You left arm is passing behind your ear. Your eyes are turned slightly downward toward your lower eyelids.

The mental focus of the pose is inward while the physical energy of the pose is downward through the feet and legs, upward and outward with the arms and hands, and on a rotational movement of the trunk to turn the belly and chest toward the ceiling. When you rotate upward, be careful not to let your left knee move forward over the arch of your left foot.

Remember that the first part of the pose is like Warrior II Pose. The second part is like Triangle Pose. As you reach out and up, allow your pelvis to

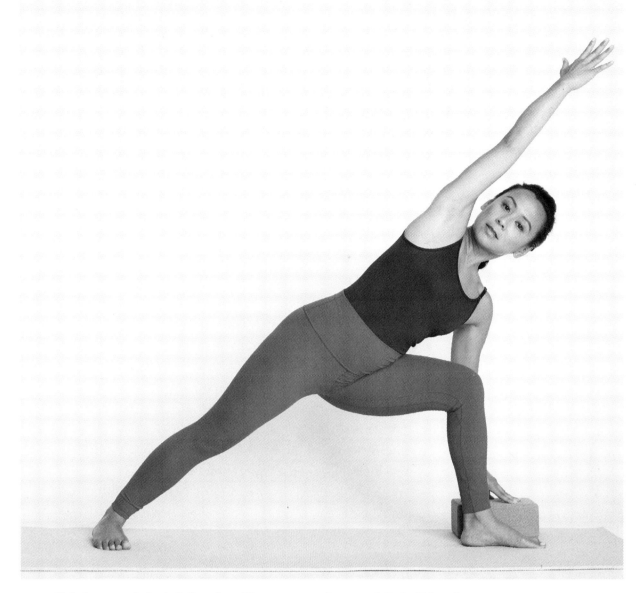

FIGURE 3.15

turn slightly toward the left foot just like you moved your pelvis in Triangle Pose when you were coming down. Do not hold the pelvis back or still; it must rotate forward and down slightly to allow the whole spine and trunk to come into a harmonious diagonal line.

You will notice that your right pelvis is slightly forward of your left pelvis, which is moving backward. This is a normal alignment of the pelvis. Remember that the pelvis is a bony ring, and if the left pelvis moves backward, the right pelvis *must* move forward. This movement is not a collapse. It is a healthy movement. Both thighs are externally rotating and abducting.

Your back will be in a normal curve. Do not tuck. If you do so, you will interfere with the ability of the pelvis to move naturally over your hip joints. Keep breathing.

To come out of the pose, turn your right palm upward toward the ceiling, and lift and press your palm and arm backward and up to lift yourself from the pose. Once you are up, take a breath, and practice the pose on the other side.

Cobra Pose

BHUJANGASANA

Special caution for these backbends: avoid these poses if you are three or more months pregnant, or if it causes pain in your lower back. You may want to consult your health-care practitioner before beginning your practice, as well as an experienced yoga teacher.

Place your folded blanket on your yoga mat and then lie on your stomach. Take a moment to make sure that your pubic bone and anterior pelvic bones are comfortable; if not, then you may want to add more padding.

Separate your legs to whatever distance you wish. Trying to hold the legs together will make it more difficult to allow the lumbosacral spine to move as it does naturally. Remember, during normal lumbar extension (backbending) the lumbar spine increases its normal curve. As it does this, it pulls the top of the sacrum, the S1 sacral segment, passively with it so that S1 moves down slightly toward the floor.

When this happens, the tailbone actually *moves upward*. This is the opposite of tucking the tailbone. Tucking the tailbone in any backbend is counter to the natural kinesiology of the lumbar spine and sacral movements. Tucking causes the lumbar to flex, not extend, as well as causing the S1 sacral segment to move up, the opposite of its normal movement in backbending. If

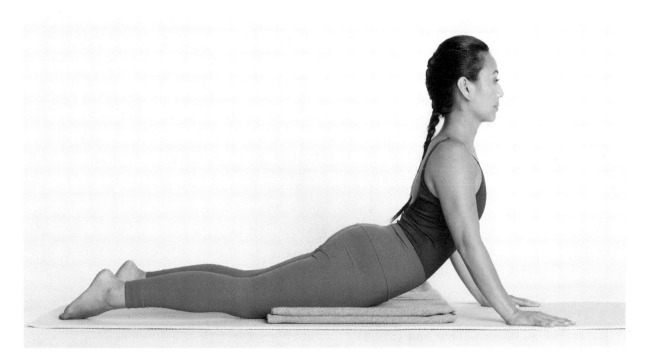

FIGURE 3.16

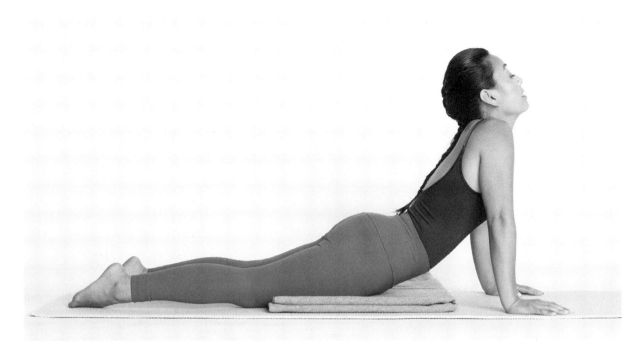

FIGURE 3.17

you tuck your tailbone in this pose you will facilitate flexion in the lumbar spine. This is exactly the *opposite* of what the pose is. *Cobra is a backbend.* Note how the model is tucking her tailbone, flattening her lumbar spine, and hanging into her shoulder joints in figure 3.17.

In order to practice Cobra as a backbend, place your hands under your shoulders, draw your shoulder blades down toward your back waist, inhale, and with an exhalation, lift up into Cobra Pose. Allow your tailbone to lift as it wants to do. This is exactly the opposite of tucking and is actually the natural movement of the back that the sacrum "wants" to do if you allow it. Imagine the very top of your sacrum pressing down toward the mat as you lift up. Be sure to draw slightly backward and upward from the back of your head and to keep your jaw parallel to the floor as you lift.

Notice how good the pose feels when you allow your legs to find their natural width in the pose, and when you let your tailbone move up so that the upper sacrum can drop, or nutate. Hold the pose for several breaths and come down. After a brief pause, repeat the pose again.

Bow Pose

DHANURASANA

Place your folded blanket on your mat for padding. Lie on your abdomen, bend your knees, and catch your ankles with your hands. Your hands should be on the outside of your ankles, with your thumbs on the outside of your ankle. With an exhalation, lift upward.

Imagine that you are lifting up in straight lines from the shoulders and the knees, rather than bending backward. Let your legs find their own distance apart. Do not try to hold them together. Allow the top of your sacrum to move firmly downward and the coccyx to move up. This facilitates nutation. Hold for several breaths, then come down. Repeat again at least one more time.

From a teaching perspective, I have noticed that students rarely complain of lower back pain in Bow Pose. I hypothesize that since you can't do this pose without nutating the sacroiliac joints and tilting the pelvis forward in an anterior tilt, there is less likelihood of discomfort.

These movements are what the body does naturally, so to be able to do the pose, there is very little need for the mind to try to "think" the backbend and thus try to tuck the tailbone.

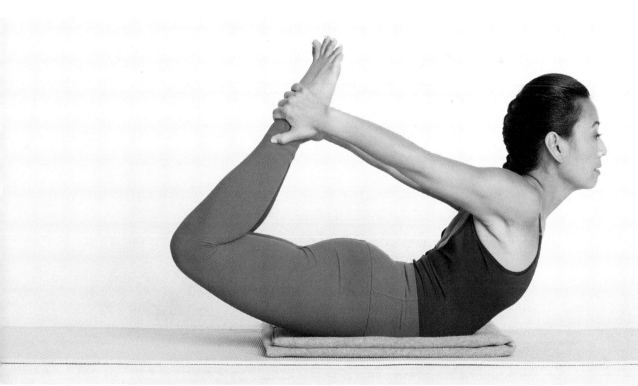

FIGURE 3.18

Camel Pose

USTRASANA

Place your folded blanket on the mat and gather two yoga blocks. Kneel, with your legs a distance apart that feels natural to you.

Put your blocks in the tallest position on the outside of your ankles. Exhaling, reach back to put your hands firmly on the blocks. It is very important that you do not tuck your tailbone in this pose. Imagine instead that your pelvis is moving forward and the pubic bone is moving downward to create an anterior pelvis tilt and thus a nutation of the sacrum and lumbar extension.

At the same time, imagine pulling your very top thighs backward. Thus, the pelvis moves forward and down and the thighs move backward. The net effect is that you will feel a strong lift in the mid-back and a lovely arch in the rest of your thoracic spine and in your lumbar. If it is comfortable, let your head hang completely backward. If this does not work for you, keep your head up. Remember to breathe a few breaths before coming out and repeating another time. Reflect on how your back feels.

Notice the model's upper back in figure 3.19. Because she allows her pelvis to move forward and tilt downward at the pubic bone (the opposite of tucking), her upper back is beautifully arched. When you are backbending, simply backbend. Do not try to tuck the tailbone to create flexion of the lumbar spine in the middle of trying to create extension there.

It is a yoga myth to think that we should tuck in a backbend. It confuses the body and overrides our natural intelligence. Your body is smarter than you are. Listen to it.

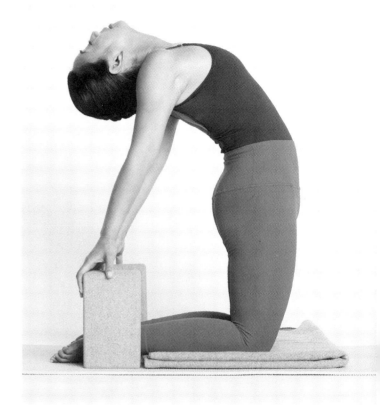

FIGURE 3.19

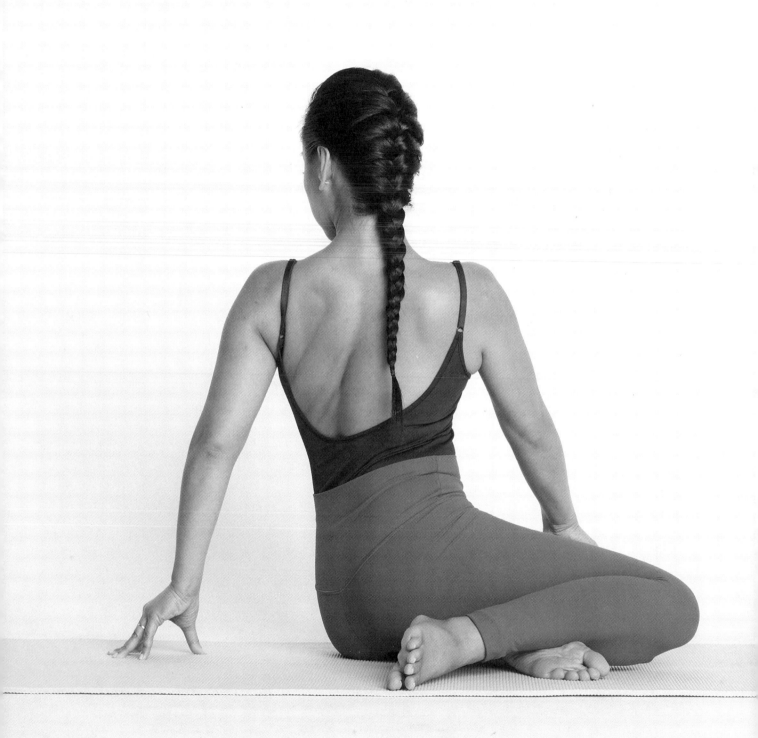

4

Free Your Pelvis and Spine, Part 2

TWISTS AND SEATED FORWARD BENDS

The pelvis is everything.

O NE DAY when I was practicing Wide-Angle Seated Forward Bend (Upavistha Konasana), I decided to stretch to one side. I firmly anchored my pelvis as I had been taught, keeping my sitting bones on the floor, then I twisted toward my left leg and reached toward my left foot with both hands.

Suddenly there was a loud and ominous "pop!" I came out of the pose immediately and over the next few days I noticed more and more discomfort around the area of my right sacroiliac joint. This discomfort prevented me from practicing twists, both seated and standing, and made my forward bend poses unpleasant as well.

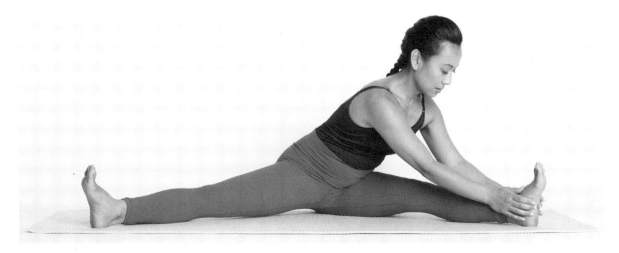

FIGURE 4.1

I finally arranged an office visit with an orthopedist, but when I showed him what I had been doing when I hurt myself, his response to me was to say, "You don't have back pain," and then he invited his nurse into the room to show her how limber I was. In hindsight, I guess he was unfamiliar with flexible people and the biomechanics of the sacrum and pelvis in yoga asana. I left without understanding what had happened and why, and just as important, how I could prevent this from ever happening again.

The pain persisted, and I was therefore left with figuring out on my own what was going on in my back. I did this by devoting my practice for the next week to only one type of pose per day. On the morning after the day I had only practiced seated twists, I was in much more pain and could hardly get out of bed. This experience reinforced in my mind that I was clearly practicing twists in a way that my body did not like. I slowly uncovered the anatomical reality of twisting and where I was going astray.

Why You Need to Know This

Often twists, especially seated twists, are taught by instructing students to "anchor the sitting bones." That is what I was doing when I was injured. I want you to understand why anchoring your sitting bones is a nonanatomical and nonfunctional way to practice twists so that you can prevent an injury like I had.

I had discovered the hard way that twists *must* be done by allowing the pelvis and sacrum to move together and not by anchoring the pelvis. Anchoring the pelvis and simultaneously twisting the vertebral column actually separates the sacroiliac joint and strains the ligamentous structures around the joint. When I practiced this new way, my pain resolved and never returned.

In this chapter, you will learn why my new approach to twists worked for me and how you can use it as well. You can prevent sustaining the injury I had, which is all too common among yoga students. This injury is based on a misunderstanding of the actual anatomical and functional relationship of the ilium of the pelvis and sacrum of the vertebral column, and what this joint needs to stay healthy and pain free.

Your Structure

Please review the "Your Anatomy in Action" section in chapter 3 before reading further. It will help you understand the material in this chapter.

In this section we will focus on the relationship between the pelvis and the sacrum. Where these two bones come together is called the sacroiliac joint (see figure 3.2 on page 40). The sacroiliac joint is made up of the union of the sacrum bone with the ilium bones on both sides of the pelvis.

The most important fact to remember about the sacroiliac joint when practicing yoga asana is that it is a joint of *stability,* not *mobility.* While there *is* a very small amount of movement allowed at the joint to facilitate walking and moving from standing to sitting and back to standing, this movement is only two to four centimeters.

This is not very much movement compared to other major joints like those of the shoulders, hips, or knees. Because the sacroiliac joint is about stability between the pelvis and the spine, it turns out that honoring this stability is the key to maintaining a happy and pain-free sacroiliac joint when you practice yoga asana.

Notice in figures 4.2 and 4.3 the many ligaments whose function it is to hold the sacrum and the pelvis together. Not only are these ligaments numerous, they are broad and strong as well.

The integrity of these ligaments is very important for maintaining the upright posture we assume, as well as for supporting the activities of daily

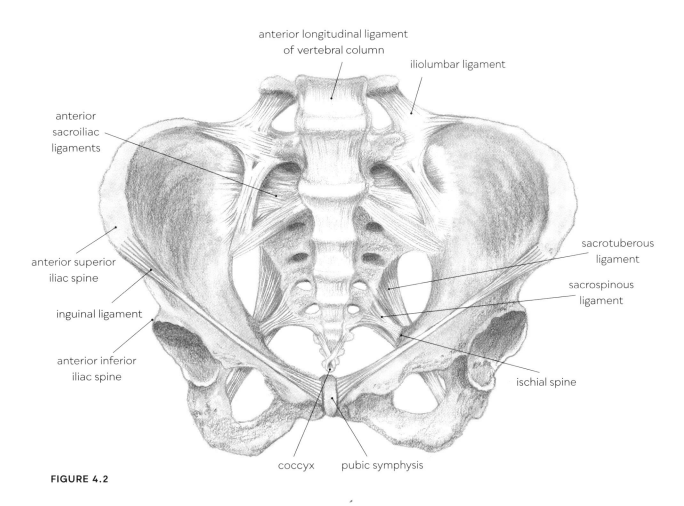

FIGURE 4.2

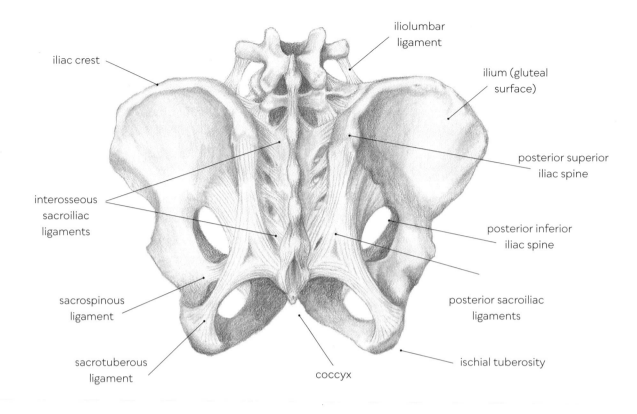

iliolumbar ligament

iliac crest

ilium (gluteal surface)

interosseous sacroiliac ligaments

posterior superior iliac spine

posterior inferior iliac spine

sacrospinous ligament

posterior sacroiliac ligaments

sacrotuberous ligament

ischial tuberosity

coccyx

FIGURE 4.3

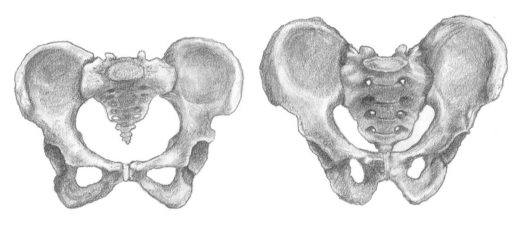

FIGURE 4.4   Female pelvis, anterior view   Male pelvis, anterior view

living that we perform, such as walking, squatting, lifting, sitting, bending, and reaching.

Besides the strength and numbers of the sacroiliac ligaments, there are other factors that can influence the stability of the sacroiliac joints. Interestingly, these are gender related. The female pelvis has a structure that is adapted for childbirth and thus is quite different in structure from the male pelvis.

The male pelvis is much narrower and smaller in shape, with a longer, narrower, and more curved sacrum, while the female pelvis is much wider at the top with a shorter, wider, flatter, more vertically oriented sacrum.

Another structural difference between the male and female pelvis is that the sacroiliac joint itself is shallower in women. When joint surfaces are deep, there is more congruence or touching between the two bones involved in the joint. For example, the hip joint is a deep joint; the acetabulum creates a well-rounded and ample surface area to receive the large and rounded head of the femur. The depth of the joint creates the increased stability that is needed at the hip joint for standing and walking. In other words, there is a great deal of congruence at the surfaces of the hip joint.

Not so with the female sacroiliac joint. In women these joint surfaces tend to be somewhat shallow. This really matters in standing because during standing the sacrum is naturally "wedged" down and against the ilium by the incumbent weight of the trunk, head, and arms. Gravity is pulling these big body parts downward and helping the sacrum stay "locked" into a more stable position against the receiving surface of the ilium.

This "wedging down" for stability is greatest when the sacrum is at an angle of about 30° to 40° and is in a diagonal line.

That means when you tuck your tailbone and thus make your sacrum vertical, or almost vertical, you are unlocking the joint, counternutating, creating less congruence, and therefore increasing instability. Tucking the tailbone in standing does not increase lower back stability; it destroys it. This action can be especially troublesome for women's lower back, hips, and sacroiliac areas since the female sacrum is already more vertically oriented than the male sacrum. Tucking for stability in standing is a yoga myth (see figure 1.5 on page 11).

There is another structural reason that the female sacroiliac joint is less stable, even with the help of the wedging mechanism created by gravity explained above. The joint surfaces in women are smaller in area where the sacrum comes together with the pelvis. Comparing the male pelvis to the female shows that there are usually three sacral segments in men that articulate with the pelvis. In women, it is more likely to be only two sacral segments that articulate with the pelvis. Remember, men have a longer sacrum than women.

The third structural reason that the female sacroiliac joint is less stable than the male has to do with the distance between the hip joints. Women have proportionally a wider distance between their hip sockets than men. When a woman steps forward with her right leg to walk, she torques her right pelvis forward and left pelvis back just like a man does. But because her hip sockets

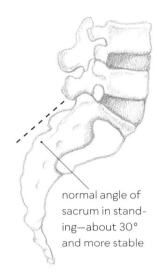

normal angle of sacrum in standing—about 30° and more stable

FIGURE 4.5
normal lumbar curve in standing

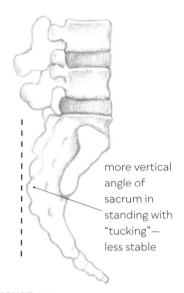

more vertical angle of sacrum in standing with "tucking"— less stable

FIGURE 4.6
"tucked" (flexed) lumbar curve in standing

are farther apart, there is more torque applied across her sacroiliac joints than there would be for a man of the same height and bone-structure size. The leverage from the front of her right pelvis diagonally across to her left sacroiliac joint in stepping forward with the right leg is simply more powerful because of the longer lever arm. The opposite is true, of course, when she steps forward with the left leg; then the right sacroiliac is slightly torqued.

Finally, women have the hormonal changes of menstruation, pregnancy, and lactation, as well as the challenge of childbirth that can affect the function of the sacroiliac ligaments. Female hormones can cause ligaments throughout the body to be more lax generally, in part to allow the pubic symphysis to spread during childbirth. When the pubic symphysis opens a bit, it stresses the ligaments holding the sacroiliac joints on the back wall of the pelvis as well.

The structural differences between the male and female pelvis, added to the hormonal differences, are the reason that about 85 percent of sacroiliac problems are to be found among women. In the next section we will learn how the sacroiliac joints can move in a healthy way in twists and forward bends.

Your Anatomy in Action

The sacroiliac ligaments function to keep the pelvis together while allowing the little bit of slippage we need, especially in walking and moving from sitting to standing and vice versa. Almost always when we move, we move our sacrum and ilium bones of the pelvis in harmony.

As discussed in chapter 3, when we backbend, the S1 sacral segment nods forward (nutation) toward the abdomen. When we forward bend, the S1 sacral segment moves backward toward the wall behind you (counternutation). Remember, these movements are small but necessary and allow us to go from standing to sitting and sitting to standing. These small movements also allow us to walk.

When we step forward with the right foot, for example, the right pelvis torques slightly forward, or in front of the left pelvis, while the left pelvis is slightly behind. The same process happens in the reverse when the left pelvis leads. Small movements make a tremendous difference in our mobility.

We need these movements when we are attempting to sit down on a chair as well. When we begin the act of sitting, the S1 segment nutates, and when we sit on the chair, the lumbar spine flexes, or rounds, and the S1 segment counternutates. You can experience this for yourself: Stand in front of a stable chair. Slowly begin to sit down and notice how you lean forward and backbend your lumbar spine. As your pelvis arrives on the seat of the chair, you now allow your lumbar spine to flex, and your S1 segment moves backward; indeed the whole sacrum moves backward from the top, or counternutates. These are normal, passive movements that follow the positioning of the lumbar spine.

The opposite occurs when you stand up. You tend to move toward the front of the seat of the chair and lean forward to create lumbar extension as you start to stand up. Your body wants to move your pelvis over your legs and feet so that your weight can be borne there. Just try standing up while keeping your lumbar spine in flexion. It simply will not work.

Let's apply the understanding of the sacrum as a joint of stability to the practice of twisting in yoga asana. Try this first: Sit on your yoga mat in Bharadvaja's Twist (Bharadvajasana) so that you are sitting mostly on your left thigh and buttock with your knees bent and legs swung to the right as in figure 4.7.

Anchor your sitting bones and pelvis. Now reach across with your right hand and place it on the outside of your left thigh just above your knee. As you exhale, try to twist without moving your pelvis; anchor from your sitting bones. You will not be able to twist very far or with most of your spine. The twist will come from the lower thoracic spine and can be unpleasant at best and painful at worst. There is a simple reason for this. When you anchor your pelvis and use your arm to pull and twist your spine, you are moving the whole spine, including the sacrum, into the twist but keeping the pelvis still.

You are in effect *twisting the spine in one direction and the pelvis in the other direction by keeping your pelvis stationary.* You are stressing the sacral ligaments, likely tending to overstretch them in an attempt to twist more, and at the same time not enjoying your pose very much. Come out of the pose.

Now try again, but this time imagine the anchor of the pose is not the pelvis and/or the sitting bones but rather the very top of the right thigh, right where the thigh becomes abdomen. Keeping your focus there, anchoring from this place, and while you are exhaling, attempt the twist. *Originate the twist by moving the pelvis over your hip joints.* Keep pressing down with your right thigh even though it will lift a little bit.

You might also enjoy imagining that your right thigh is stretching outward strongly away from your pelvis and is getting longer while it moves away from the hip socket.

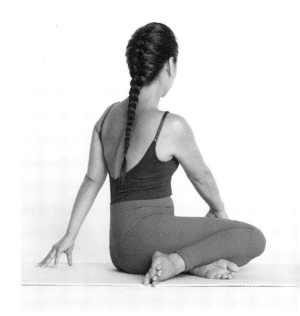

FIGURE 4.7

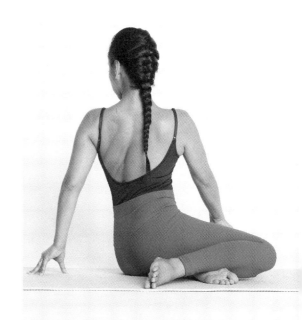

FIGURE 4.8

Your right buttock might lift up a little bit, but that is actually part of the pose as long as you are moving the hip sockets of the pelvis around and over the femoral heads and thus creating the movement from the hip joints. In other words, the pelvis is moving *with* the spinal column, not in the opposite direction. Now try this new way of twisting in Bharadvaja's Twist to the other side.

What you have done by twisting in this manner is to shift your idea of where you anchor the pose. Instead of anchoring the sitting bones and pelvis, you are anchoring your legs. Remember, you create many other poses through the hip joints, especially all forward bends and standing poses. And in these poses you are anchoring from and with your legs. Do the same thing in twists.

Why does twisting this way protect the sacroiliac joint? Because it keeps the pelvis and sacrum moving together. The key to healthy movement in twisting during asana practice and in daily life is simple: move from your pelvis.

When you anchor your pelvis in a twist, you are in effect moving your pelvis *out* of the twist. At the same time, your sacrum is being pulled by the spine to move *into* the twist. Separating the sacrum from the ilium is the definition of sacroiliac dysfunction.

The "separation" of the joint in this manner is what causes the pain, and sometimes swelling, around the joint. The habitual stretching of the sacral ligaments in asana usually overstretches them, creating laxity in the joint and setting you up for a chronic condition in which the ilium and sacrum are not correctly positioned in a stable way and that creates sacroiliac pain.

That is exactly what I did to myself in the anecdote at the beginning of this chapter. I sat in a Wide-Angle Seated Forward Bend, anchored my pelvis, and used my arms to pull my sacrum and spine over my right leg. That injured the soft tissues around my sacroiliac joint and overstretched my sacral ligaments. I had nagging symptoms for a long time until I finally learned to move my pelvis and my sacrum together at all times.

And this includes during activities of daily living. Begin to notice the relationship of your sacrum and pelvis not only in your asana practice but also when you are going through your day. When you reach across your body to pick something up, are you letting your pelvis go with your spine? When you sleep on your side, are you keeping a harmonious relationship between your sacrum and ilium, or are you lying in such a way as to pull your spine forward and leave your pelvis behind?

If you bring this principle of creating and maintaining stability between your pelvis and sacrum into your practice and during your day, you will be much less likely to have sacroiliac problems. So simple.

Attentive Practice

The sacroiliac joint is actually easy to understand. It is important that as you practice the poses in this section, you remember to move your sacrum and pelvis together, so that you are following the body's natural wisdom and preventing injury at the same time.

CAUTIONS

Avoid these poses if you have lower back pain, especially if you have diagnosed disc disease, sacroiliac dysfunction, or any concerns about twisting or forward bending.

PROPS NEEDED

- Nonslip yoga mat
- One or two yoga blocks
- One or two yoga blankets

Revolved Triangle Pose
PARIVRTTA TRIKONASANA

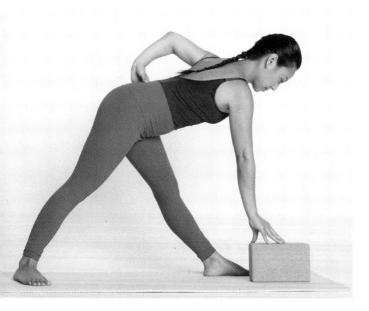

FIGURE 4.9

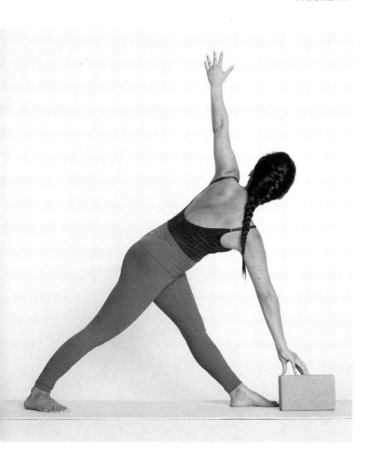

FIGURE 4.10

This is a twisted version of the Extended Triangle Pose that was discussed in chapter 3. To begin, step onto your mat and place your feet two-and-a-half to three-and-a-half feet apart. Place your block on the arch side of your left foot. Start with the block just even with the arch, but be willing to move it forward as needed. Just how far forward the block is when you are in the pose will be determined in part by the length of your trunk. Try a few different block placements to find the most comfortable distance.

Turn and face your left leg. Turn your left foot to the left, a little past 90°. Turn your right foot inward so it is facing about half the way forward. Your right toes are now facing almost forward in the same direction as your left toes. You may also enjoy moving your left foot to the right a few inches so that you feel more stable in this stance. Experiment a bit to find the right distance for you.

Now turn your pelvis toward your front foot so you are facing your left leg. Raise your arms over your head as you inhale. Bend forward, placing your right fingers firmly on the block and drawing your left elbow upward toward the ceiling as you exhale. Let your whole trunk and pelvis turn with you. Slowly straighten your arm toward the ceiling. Look straight ahead of you rather than upward; this is easier for the neck.

With several slow and natural exhalations, gently move your pelvis and your trunk forward toward your right arm. Lift up through your arm while stretching and pushing downward at the same time. Do not let most of your weight fall onto your block but rather imagine that you are stretching in two directions at once, so the emphasis is on lifting up, not on hanging down into the bottom arm.

Create the twist from the pelvis moving forward over your femoral heads. Make sure that your right pelvis is closer to the ground than your left. But the right pelvis is not in front of or behind the left pelvis. Do not keep your sacrum parallel to the ground. If you do so, you will be stressing the sacroiliac joint by anchoring the pelvis and pulling the spine away from it. Moving from the pelvis will allow the twist to be deeper, easier, and more satisfying.

Then imagine a backbend in your lumbar spine and a twist in your thoracic spine so that your left shoulder blade is directly in a vertical line over your right shoulder blade. Slightly backbend in the mid-thoracic spine as well.

When you are in the position try this breathing, which should be avoided if you are pregnant: Inhale, then exhale completely, and before inhaling again, twist from deep in the pelvis as if your lower belly organs are leading the twisting movement. Think of moving your belly organs around from facing the floor to facing the ceiling. The breath is totally out while you are doing this short twisting action. Once you are twisted, breathe softly and try one more time by exhaling completely and twisting after the exhalation is complete.

Twists are healthiest when they originate from the pelvis, allowing the sacrum to remain in harmony with the pelvis. You will have a deeper and more satisfying twist when you let the pelvis rotate around the hip joints and involve the pelvis completely.

To come out of the pose, exhale as you bring your left hand down, then bring your pelvis into a level position like a forward bend, with both hands down to the floor or your ankle. Inhale as you come up, maintaining the normal curves of the vertebral column as you do so. Repeat the pose on the other side.

Remember that in Revolved Triangle Pose *do not try to keep your sacrum and pelvis level.* This holds the sacrum back while the rest of your spine is pulling it forward. If you twist this way, the twist will feel very incomplete. There will be no pressure on the abdominal organs, which I believe is one of the most important parts of twisting.

The pressure caused by the twist, whether it's a standing or a seated one, squeezes the organs. When you untwist, the organs resume their natural shape. One way to know if you are practicing your twists from your organs and not just your spine is that you will feel a sense of heat in the pose and/or when you come out. Twists are warming because I believe that they help to stimulate and move your *apana* energy in the abdomen.

If you practice this pose by keeping your sacrum and back pelvis parallel to the floor, you will not produce this healthy pressure on your abdominal organs, and in my opinion, will not get the full benefit of the pose. In addition, by keeping the sacrum and back pelvis parallel to the floor, you are keeping the pelvis still but pulling the sacrum forward, which stresses the sacroiliac joint.

Seated Twist

MARICHYASANA III

This is one of the most common twists taught in modern asana. Begin by sitting on your mat and bending your left knee. Place your left heel *exactly* in line with your left sitting bone. Allow some space between your left foot and your inner groin.

If you place your foot so it is touching your inner right thigh, this will cause your left knee to fall outward a bit, thus changing the relationship of your femur in your hip joint and making it more difficult to twist. Your shin should be vertical, so be sure to bend your knee just enough, so your shin is neither too close nor too far away from your left thigh.

If you feel like you are falling backward, try moving your heel a little farther out and/or sit on the corner of one or two folded blankets. Sitting on the corner will allow your pelvis to be lifted up and your legs to drop down around the edges of the blanket.

The next step is the most important one in the pose. With an exhalation, slide your right leg and right pelvis forward. Your right sitting bone will now be several inches forward of your left sitting bone. This action is a movement created from the hip joints.

Notice that you are already twisted a bit and perhaps even facing your inner left thigh. Make sure that your pelvis is twisted with the spine. This will mean that your pelvis and sacrum are both twisting together, which is exactly the action that will protect your sacroiliac joint.

Hug your left leg with your right arm. Keep your breathing free and make all your movements on an exhalation. Shift your weight so about 90 percent of it, or more, is on the left sitting bone and the right buttock is barely touching the floor.

Use your left hand behind you to propel yourself forward. Move your rib cage horizontally forward by rolling your pubic bone down toward the floor. Make sure that your weight is still on your left sitting bone and the right buttock is barely touching the floor. Keep stretching out from the right leg. Making sure that you have not moved your left foot, press your weight down through your left tibia onto your foot.

Inhale and exhale completely so that your abdominal muscles are contracting and the air is mostly out of your lungs. (Do not use this breathing technique if you are pregnant.) After the exhalation, when the lungs are empty, twist from your pelvis. Think of moving your belly organs around the spine into the twist as you did in Revolved Triangle Pose. Repeat this breath several times as you continue to twist in the same direction.

You may find that you want to place your right upper arm across your left knee or thigh, but it is not necessary. If you do place your elbow across your leg, keep your elbow slightly bent to avoid hyperextending the elbow joint. You may also enjoy hugging your left leg to facilitate the pose as the model is demonstrating in figure 4.11 below.

Make sure that each time you attempt to twist a little farther, you are using your pelvis to originate the movement and that the weight stays on your left sitting bone. Press strongly down on your left foot as if you were going to stand up on that foot. Remember that the left tibia is the anchor of the pose, not the sitting bones.

Hold the twist for several breaths, then slowly come out of it. Be sure to practice the pose on the right side, too.

It is highly likely that you twisted farther than usual, and that the twist felt more intense and more satisfying at the same time. You also may experience heat in your midsection or in your chest and face. I believe that this heat is caused by the squeezing effect on the abdominal organs that I mentioned earlier, and as I proposed, this heat represents the release of apana energy that is being dispersed throughout the abdomen and chest. Some students feel the almost overwhelming desire to lie down after practicing each side of the twist. By all means, do so. This allows the belly organs to expand after the squeezing effect.

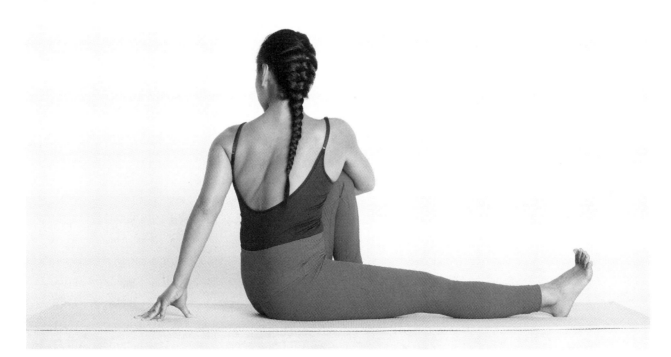

FIGURE 4.11

Head-to-Knee Pose
JANU SIRSASANA

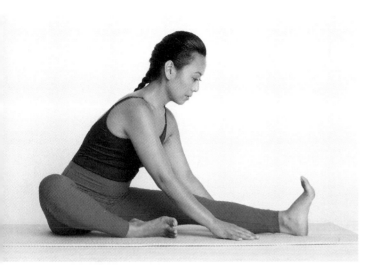

This forward bend is a popular one; however, this does not mean that it is easy. I rarely teach this to beginning students because they understretch the legs and overwork the lower back. I would suggest that if you have tight hamstrings (back of the thigh muscles), very tight hips, or lower back pain, you should skip this pose until those conditions improve. Instead, work on the traditional standing poses.

To practice, sit on your mat with both legs straight out in front of you. Inhale, and with an exhalation, bring your right foot near your groin, but slightly out in a diagonal line.

The first thing to observe is how high your right thigh and right knee are from the floor. In order to proceed, they need to be very close to the floor. If you are almost there, you might enjoy propping your knee up with a blanket, but only for three or so inches, no higher. If your knee is higher, please be very careful with this pose.

Additionally, in order to protect your lower back and gain the most benefit from the pose, you must be able to sit in front of your sitting bones. If this is not yet possible, skip this pose and work on standing poses, especially standing forward bends to create more flexibility in your hamstrings and hip rotators.

If your right knee is on the floor, or close to it, proceed. Notice how this pose is a kind of twist. Your right pelvis is farther back than your left, so in effect when you are sitting there, you are actually sitting in a slight right twist.

The challenge of the pose is to bring your right pelvis into the forward bend evenly with your left. This means that there is more action from the right pelvis than the left, because the right pelvis must move farther forward in order to keep the pelvis even. Just reaching and stretching forward without concentrating on bringing the right pelvis forward with you will torque the sacroiliac joint as you go down.

The right leg, even though it is bent, is the active leg in this pose. The left leg receives the action of the forward bend, which the right leg and pelvis create. The right leg *anchors* the pose when you press firmly down at the root of your right hip joint. The right pelvis *creates* the action by lifting up and rolling over the stationary right femur at its root. If you do not concentrate more on the right pelvis than the left by moving it over the femur as you bend forward, you are stressing the sacroiliac joint.

Inhale, and exhaling, turn your body, from the pelvis, toward the left. Take your right pelvis with you in this slight twisting movement. Reach down with your right hand and catch the outside of your left knee or ankle. This action must be done by tipping your pelvis forward or there is great stress put on the structures of your lower back.

Sometimes sitting up on the corner of a folded blanket or two can help you tip your pelvis. Note the position of the model's pelvis. Focus on the alignment of the pose, and the range of movement will come over time. Alignment before range. You are much less likely to pull a muscle or injure yourself in some other way if you focus on alignment first and range second.

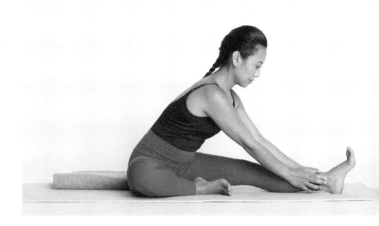

FIGURE 4.13

If you can go farther down and still originate the move from the pelvis, then reach both hands down past your left foot and hold your right wrist with your left hand. This way of holding will help you keep your arms and knees straight.

Align your breastbone with the inside of your left thigh. Do not move your breastbone over your thigh. Practicing this way may facilitate a delicious stretch over your back right waist. I like to practice so that my stretch sensation in the pose is equally shared with my right hamstrings and my back right waist.

Keep breathing softly, drop your head so it is in line with your spine, and hold for ten breaths. Slowly come up by using your arms to help, and practice on the other side. It is very important to remember that as you come down slowly into the pose, the movement is mostly coming from the right side of your body: the right hip joint and the right pelvis. The pelvis leads the way. When practiced this way, you will probably feel that equal stretch in your hamstrings and in your right back waist mentioned above. When you move the sacrum and the pelvis together, the sacroiliac joint will remain your friend.

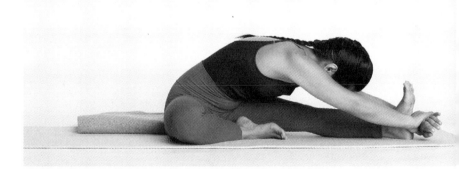

FIGURE 4.14

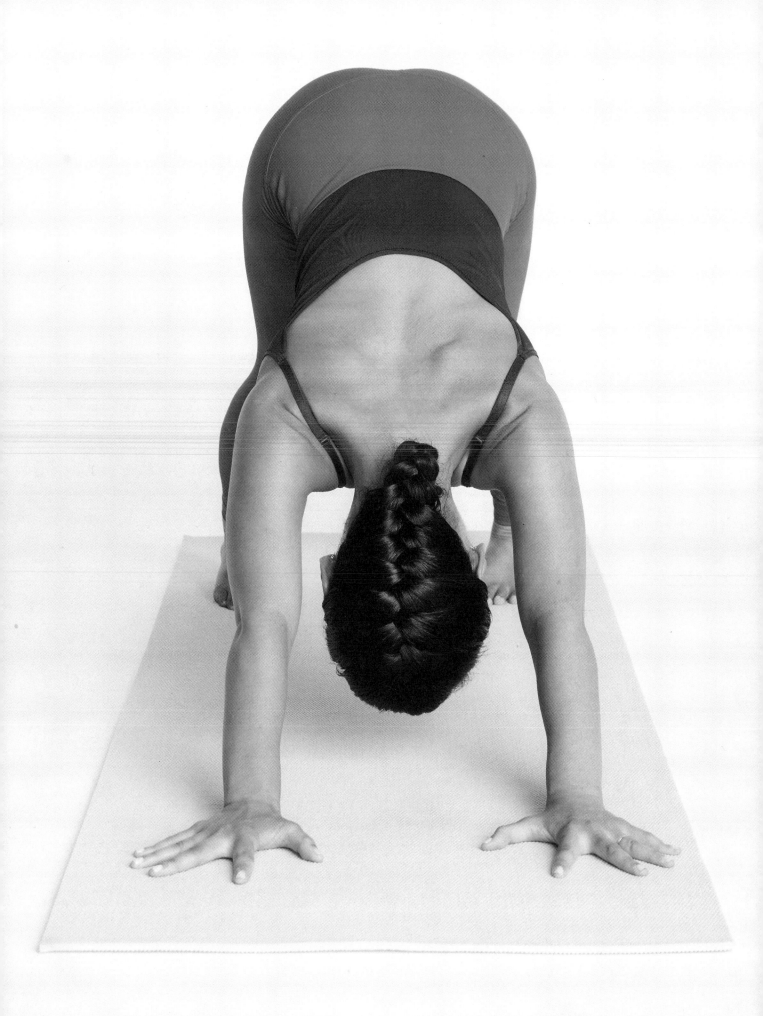

5

Fly from Your Wings

WHEN TO MOVE YOUR SHOULDER BLADES AND WHEN NOT TO

The shoulder blade is the root of the shoulder joint.

Years ago, I was teaching a workshop for teachers that was specifically focused on the anatomy of the shoulder joint. As part of this workshop, students were also learning how to apply this anatomical knowledge in a practical manner to create healthy shoulder movements in Downward-Facing Dog Pose (Adho Mukha Svanasana) and other common poses involving the shoulder joint.

Unbeknownst to me, participating in this class was a teacher who was suffering from chronic shoulder pain when she was in the pose. She was using her shoulder joint in the exact *opposite* way from what the anatomical structure of the joint suggests it be used, because she had been frequently instructed to do so in this pose. She had had shoulder pain in Downward-Facing Dog Pose for years, and as I looked at her pose, I could guess that she was suffering without her saying anything.

I suggested that she rotate her upper arms in the opposite direction from what she was doing, to release the scapula and let it rotate and move toward her hands. When she did so, the pain she had had for years almost immediately disappeared. I was to learn later from her that not only did the pain disappear right then in the class, but it never came back in the pose as long as she followed the suggestions she was given. Upon returning home, she shared the wonderful news with her family that her shoulder pain was gone. It was a dramatic and very welcome result for her. Partly because of what happened in that workshop, we soon became colleagues and friends. She is the author of the foreword to this book as well.

I have heard similar stories from many other students for years. Additionally, what I have learned from my own personal practice, from my training to become a physical therapist, and from what I have seen in decades of teaching has convinced me that understanding the structure and function of your shoulder joint can prevent injury and alleviate discomfort.

My request of you as a reader is that you study this chapter and then begin to experiment with a new approach to using your shoulder joints in Downward-Facing Dog Pose and other asana involving these joints.

Why You Need to Know This

I believe that there is a fundamentally flawed understanding widely held by many yoga teachers and students about how the shoulder joint actually moves in asana. That is why I often teach workshops that focus exclusively on the natural and healthy movements of the shoulder joints.

I really want yoga teachers to "live in" and teach from the basis of anatomical reality when instructing shoulder movements. I want you, as a student of yoga asana, to know this as well, so that you can keep yourself safe in any yoga class.

Living in harmony with anatomical reality means that when we teach and practice, we allow the healthy biomechanics of shoulder movement to spontaneously occur. We follow the natural movements of the shoulder joints and do not impose an intellectual dictum on our shoulder movements. In effect, we need to "listen to our shoulder joints" rather than "tell our shoulder joints what to do" in asana. Remember, your body is smarter than you are.

We will learn about the specific anatomy and normal movements of the shoulder joint in this chapter. I especially hope you will study well the two sections titled "Your Structure" and "Your Anatomy in Action." One of the things you will learn there, for example, is that turning your upper arm outward into external rotation at the end range of flexion in Downward-Facing Dog Pose while holding your scapula down can and often does impinge the supraspinatus tendon between the scapula and the head of your humerus. This can contribute to pain, supraspinatus tendonitis, and tears in the tendon. (More on this later.)

Learning a new way to practice that honors your body's natural structure and intelligence when moving can free up not only your Downward-Facing Dog Pose but other poses involving the shoulder joint as well. No doubt this new way of moving your shoulder joints will also make your practice safer and more satisfying at the same time.

Your Structure

As the quote at the beginning of this chapter implies, to understand the shoulder joint, one must first get to know the scapula. The scapula is the key to how we move the entire upper extremity, which is made up of the humerus, clavicle, sternum, radius and ulna (forearm bones), the carpals (wristbones), the metacarpals (hand bones), and the phalanges (finger bones).

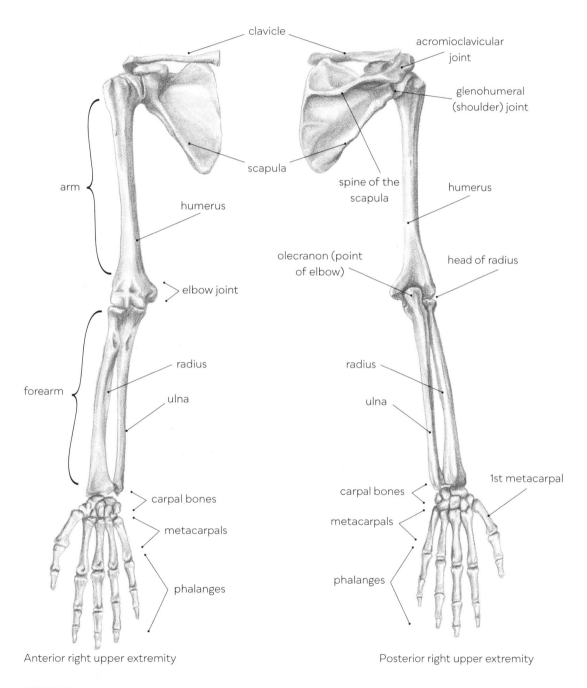

Anterior right upper extremity

Posterior right upper extremity

FIGURE 5.1

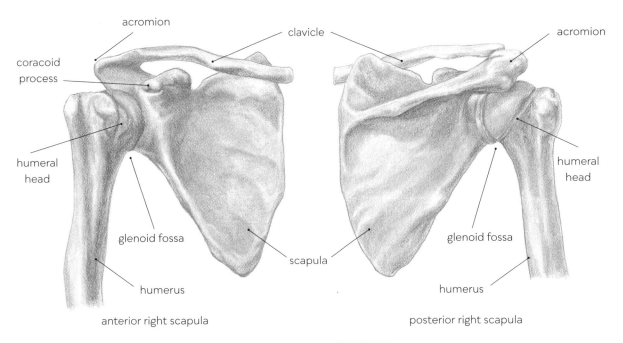

acromion

coracoid
process

humeral
head

glenoid fossa

humerus

anterior right scapula

FIGURE 5.2

clavicle

acromion

humeral
head

glenoid fossa

scapula

humerus

posterior right scapula

FIGURE 5.3

The scapula bone is in the shape of a pyramid standing on its head, and it is curved to fit snugly and perfectly over the ribs. It is actually a joint and is called the scapulothoracic joint. Please note figures 5.2 and 5.3, which point out the various bony landmarks and structures of the scapula and humerus. The junction of the scapula and the humerus is what we might call the "true shoulder joint." It is the ball-and-socket part of the joint and is known as the glenohumeral joint (named for the cavity on the lateral scapula that forms the socket of the shoulder joint and for the head of the arm bone that fits into that socket).

Besides connecting with the humerus, the scapula also connects on the front of the body to the clavicle. The other end of the clavicle connects to the sternum. This group of joints must all work together in harmony to allow for normal and pain-free movement in the shoulder joint.

Notice the relationship between the tendon of the supraspinatus and the head of the humerus in figure 5.4.

It is possible to move the humerus in such a way as to entrap this tendon between the acromion and the humeral head (see figure 5.5). This entrapment will be explained further in the next section, but basically entrapment occurs in part when the humerus is externally rotated instead of internally rotated at the very end of flexion and abduction. Entrapment also occurs when the shoulder blades are not allowed to move but rather are purposively held still in flexion and abduction.

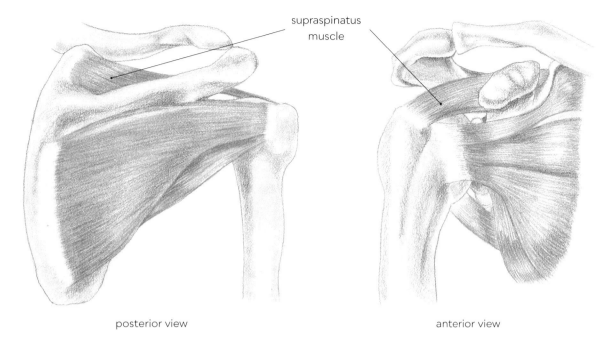

supraspinatus
muscle

posterior view

anterior view

FIGURE 5.4

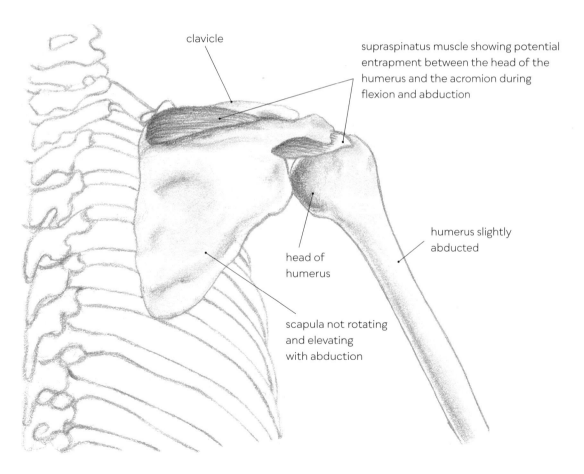

clavicle

supraspinatus muscle showing potential
entrapment between the head of the
humerus and the acromion during
flexion and abduction

head of
humerus

humerus slightly
abducted

scapula not rotating
and elevating
with abduction

FIGURE 5.5

Your Anatomy in Action

How can we avoid the entrapment of the supraspinatus tendon when practicing yoga? By letting the scapula move freely when we take the upper extremity into both full flexion and full abduction.

Note the model in the figures on the next page. In figure 5.6 she is holding the scapula still and even pulling it down toward the waist as many students are instructed to do when they take their arms overhead. In figure 5.7, the model is now allowing the scapula to swing out and away from the vertebral column, thus rotating the inferior angle outward to the side body as she brings her arms over her head. Note the different positions of her shoulder blades in these two photos.

If your shoulder is functioning well and is pain free, try this. Stand up and abduct one of your arms out to your side about a foot. Move slowly and notice that your scapula does not move very much at the beginning of the movement. Now continue to move the arm up, and you will immediately feel the scapula beginning to rotate and elevate if you do not consciously interfere with it doing so.

This rotation and elevation is a normal part of flexion (the arm moving to the front of your body and up all the way) and abduction of the shoulder joint. This scapular movement happens naturally from the innate intelligence of the body both in abduction and flexion. In fact, this rotation and elevation of the scapula is extremely important in flexion and abduction to prevent injury to the shoulder joint. If your shoulder health permits, try abducting your arm all the way up so your arm is over your head without moving your scapula.

It is not possible. Undoubtedly you feel stuck about halfway up if you impede the scapula from rotating. Now try abduction again and notice the point where your scapula starts to move. Let it rotate. Let it elevate. This is what the scapula was "designed" to do in abduction and flexion. This is anatomical reality.

The rotation and elevation of the scapula during flexion and abduction is part of what is called the glenohumeral or scapulohumeral rhythm. The scapulae are moved by several muscles, including the serratus anterior and the upper trapezius. Furthermore, the head of the humerus is moved in the scapular socket by four muscles: the supraspinatus, infraspinatus, teres minor, and subscapularis. These four muscles are involved in positioning the head of the arm bone in the socket during this rhythm and make flexion and abduction possible.

To feel the normal scapular movement in another way, imagine you are reaching up for something you really want that is up on a high shelf. Focus on what you want and really stretch up without "thinking" the movement. Let

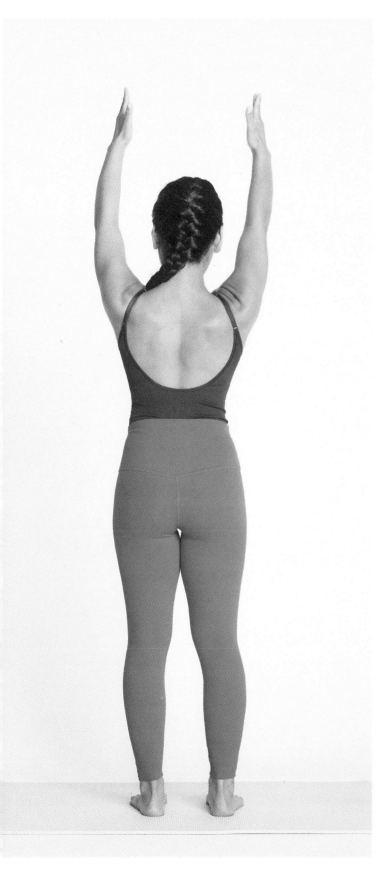

FIGURE 5.6

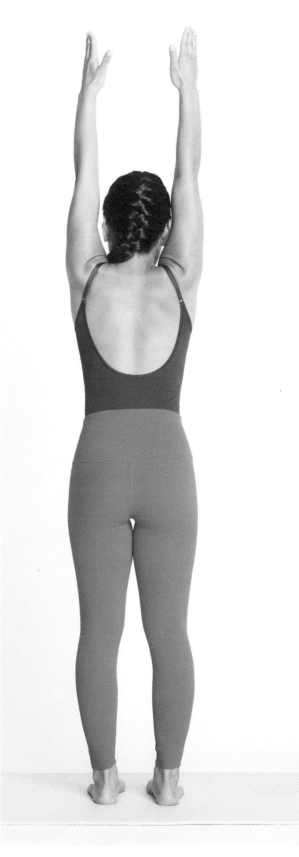

FIGURE 5.7

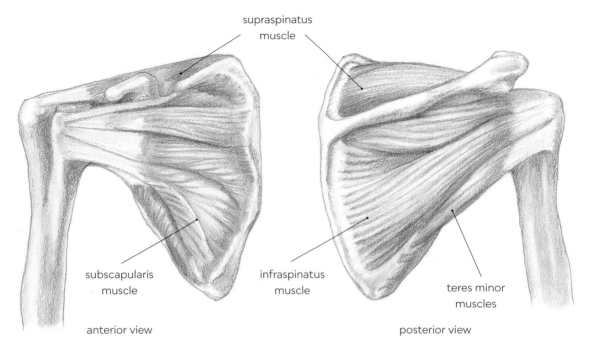

supraspinatus muscle

subscapularis muscle

infraspinatus muscle

teres minor muscles

anterior view

posterior view

FIGURE 5.8
Rotator cuff muscles

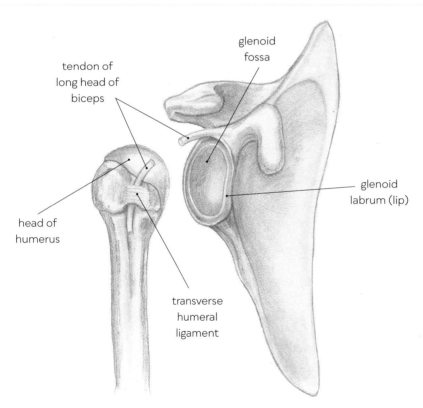

tendon of long head of biceps

glenoid fossa

glenoid labrum (lip)

head of humerus

transverse humeral ligament

FIGURE 5.9

your scapula elevate. Let the outside or lateral border of your scapula really move up. Feel how much freedom you have to move in your shoulder joint when your mind is not interfering with what the scapula "wants" to do naturally.

Why does it feel so much easier and so much better to move this way? Look at figure 5.9. Note the glenoid fossa, the curved receiving hollow on the lateral scapula where the head of the humerus joins the scapula to create the true shoulder joint.

When your scapula swings out from the spine in rotation and elevates in flexion and abduction, your glenoid fossa turns and faces upward, like a hollow of a cup faces upward when you hold it. When your arm is hanging down by your side, the glenoid fossa is facing out to the side. But when the scapula rotates and elevates freely, not only does it bring the glenoid into an upward-facing position, but it also allows the head of the humerus to move out from under the shelf of the acromion, and thus the humerus does not entrap the supraspinatus tendon.

I call the acromion the "roof" of the shoulder joint. Letting your scapula rotate outward and move upward, so that the glenoid is turned toward the sky, is critical for the health of the supraspinatus tendon that crosses under the acromion and attaches to the head of the humerus. Thus scapular rotation creates space between the "roof" of the shoulder joint and humeral head for the supraspinatus tendon to be free. This happens naturally if you do not interfere with the movement.

External rotation of the humerus is also required for both abduction and flexion to be normal. However, when one reaches full shoulder flexion like in Downward-Facing Dog Pose and Warrior II Pose, continuing to rotate externally will now begin to make the joint less free. At the end range of flexion, it is time to internally rotate to neutral where you will find maximal joint configuration. We will practice this principle in the next section, "Attentive Practice."

Finally, there are two other parts of the glenohumeral rhythm besides humeral rotation and scapular rotation and elevation that are necessary to allow full flexion and abduction. These are a longitudinal rotation of the clavicle and the extension, or backbending, of the thoracic spine.

To feel the rotation of the collarbone, let your left arm hang down by your side. With two fingers of your right hand, gently hold your collarbone at the place it feels most prominent in the front of your body.

Now abduct your left arm and feel how the clavicle rotates inwardly, or in toward your body. This happens because the clavicle is attached directly to the scapula at the acromion. So as the scapula moves, the clavicle is pulled up at the lateral or outer side and rotates passively to do this. In other words,

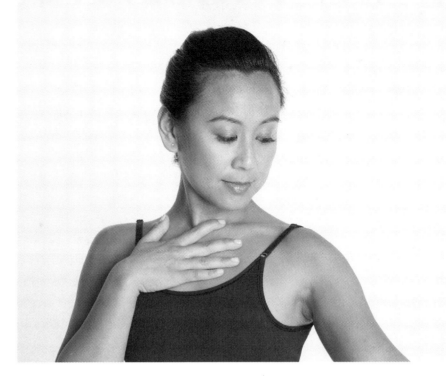

FIGURE 5.10

there is no muscle that rotates the clavicle. The clavicle is passively pulled upward at the lateral side by the rotation and elevation of the scapula.

Interestingly, some students can't fully flex or abduct the shoulder joint because their upper back is too stiff, not because the glenohumeral joint is dysfunctional. The normal rounded shape of the thoracic spine must reverse into slight extension—a backbend—in order to allow the scapula to move over the rib cage. Thus, the thoracic spine can affect the movement of the scapula as it rotates and elevates when we flex or abduct the arm. If the superior thoracic spine from T1 to T4 cannot backbend, flexion and abduction will not be normal.

Try one last experiment. Proceeding slowly and with care, let your upper back round forward as when you are slumping. Now hold your back in this slumping position and try to abduct or to flex your shoulder joint. Be very slow and careful and do not force it. Likely you will feel limited as you attempt to do these two movements, and that limitation probably feels like a "bony block" in the shoulder joint. That is because *it is a bony block* in the shoulder joint; the head of the humerus is hitting against the acromion. This is not what the shoulder joint "wants" to do.

Now try abduction and flexion by letting your upper back arch naturally and freely as you move your arm over your head. This is what your body is made to do, structurally and functionally. Moving in this manner respects the body's innate intelligence.

If you experiment with living in anatomical reality and letting your shoulder blades move in full abduction and full flexion, my guess is that you will be happier and your shoulder joint will move with freedom and joy.

In asana practice, however, we do not just need our shoulders to move freely; sometimes we need our shoulder joints to be held still in order to create stability, for example when we do poses with weight on our arms. In these poses we are creating a very different relationship with gravity than we are when we take the arms over the head or out to the side in standing.

When we do poses that demand strength and stability from our shoulders, the scapula needs to be held firmly against the ribs and trunk. In a posture like Plank Pose (Chaturanga Dandasana), we do not move or rotate the scapula. We will experiment with this principle in the "Attentive Practice" section.

MAIN POINTS TO REMEMBER FROM THIS CHAPTER

→ The position of the scapula, as well as how it moves, is the priority focus in any asana practice involving the upper body.

→ Allow the scapula to elevate and rotate naturally in flexion and abduction of the shoulder joint.

→ The scapula needs to be held firmly against the rib cage and back and does not rotate during poses in which the arms are bearing all, or a significant portion, of your body weight.

Attentive Practice

The shoulder is probably the most complicated joint in your body. Move with care during these practices and make friends with your shoulders.

CAUTIONS

Be cautious when practicing these shoulder movements, especially if you already have pain in your shoulder joints. This type of pain is not a healthy pain. If a movement causes discomfort in a joint, you may want to consider a consultation with your health-care provider before continuing.

PROPS NEEDED

- Nonslip yoga mat

- Two-inch-wide yoga belt, at least four feet long

Warrior I Pose

VIRABHADRASANA I

Step onto your mat. Separate your feet so they're about three-and-a-half feet apart. This distance will depend on the length of your legs. Don't worry; you can adjust it as you begin to practice the pose.

To practice to the left, turn your right foot inward about 45° and your left foot slightly out so your left leg is externally rotated. Make sure that your pelvis is turned toward the left leg.

While you are inhaling, lift your arms out to the side and up all the way. When you do this, be sure to elevate your shoulder blades as you lift your arms. In order for you to get your arms straight up, your shoulder blades need to rotate and lift.

Here's an important note about this action: you may have been taught specifically to keep your shoulder blades down to "release the neck" in the pose. Yet, as we learned in the sections above, the scapula must lift up in order to afford us full flexion. The scapular elevators are the levator scapulae muscle and the upper fibers of the trapezius muscle. Both muscles work together to elevate the scapula at the end of the range of flexion like you are doing in this pose. (Remember, this elevation also occurs during abduction.)

Using the scapular elevators to elevate the scapula is normal. What we want to avoid, however, is tensing the front throat when we do this elevation. "Lifting" from the front of the body is *not* a healthy elevation of the scapula.

Make sure that you are using the muscles in your back body to elevate and rotate your scapula to allow yourself full flexion of the shoulder joints. One way to know that you are doing this is to notice how it feels. Once your arms are up and stretching toward the ceiling, do you feel that you could keep reaching forever? Do you feel that your arms are "growing" up and out of your belly and pelvis? Is there any sense of stretch in your belly? Do you feel the joy of really letting the body take over the movement? Then it is likely you are honoring the natural intelligence of your body and letting your scapulae do what they do best: rotate and elevate in flexion and abduction.

Remember to breathe as you stretch upward. Now bend your left knee over your left little toe. Imagine that your lower body is connected to the earth, and your upper body is flying toward the heavens. Stay present between these two opposite directions.

As much as possible, make sure that your left thigh is parallel to the floor, that your right leg is actively pressing back and down, and your heel and outer back right foot are grounded. Let your lower back arch, as is demonstrated by the model in figure 5.11.

Your pelvis will tip forward when you allow a natural bend in your back. Remember, to take your arms into full flexion; you need to backbend your thoracic spine; let your lumbar arch as well.

If you wish, and if your neck will allow it, you also may like to let your head drop backward. To do this, bring your arms in front of your head slightly, and while breathing softly, press your palms together. Notice how your upper chest muscles are active.

Keep your arms in an exactly vertical line. Perhaps a teacher or fellow yoga student can tell you when your arms are indeed vertical. Do not let your arms reach or fall backward. They stay firmly in front of your chest and head slightly and in a vertical line. Visualize your arms being pulled upward and inward toward each other. They are your "lifeline" in the pose. Brace yourself strongly on your right leg, and while exhaling, let your head and neck rest back.

Be sure that you do this movement with your whole neck first and then your head. Sometimes I have seen students attempt this movement by first pushing their chin forward, then crunching the back of their head down onto the neck to look up at the ceiling. What happens when you start this movement by pushing the chin forward is that you actually flex the cervical spine; the only part that actually backbends is the skull on the neck, using only the upper cervical vertebrae. It is similar to the dynamics of a forward head posture (see figure 1.3 on page 6), which is to be avoided. If you are backbending the neck, let the head hang off the neck as if you could easily look at the floor behind you once you are in full extension. Keep moving the arms up and inward. And keep breathing.

Turn your eyes downward to rest on your lower eyelids; do not look up. Soften your jaw, cheeks, and tongue. You are moving toward earth and heaven and creating a beautiful shape that balances the yielding of the chest and back, and the strength of the legs and the arms. You are a "warrior" yielding into all the strength you possess.

Take a few breaths in the pose, then lift your head, straighten your knee as you inhale, and lower your arms with an exhalation. When you are ready, repeat on the right side.

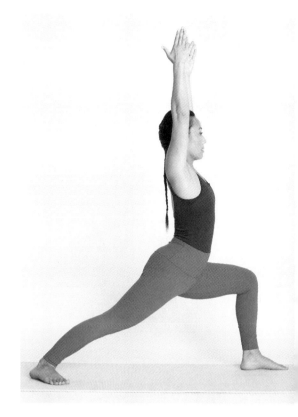

FIGURE 5.11

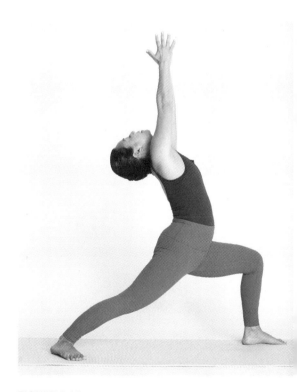

FIGURE 5.12

Downward-Facing Dog Pose

ADHO MUKHA SVANASANA

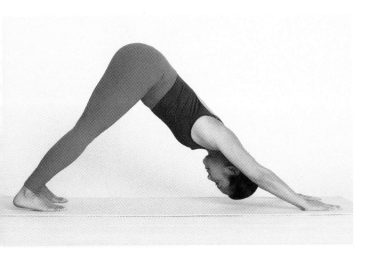

FIGURE 5.13

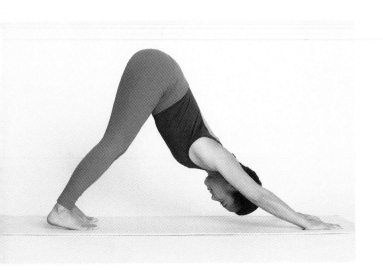

FIGURE 5.14

Step onto your mat and get down on your hands and knees. Let your head hang down and take a few moments to place your hands so that your middle fingers point straight forward.

Push your thumbs and index fingers firmly into the floor. They make up the "brain of the hand" in this pose. Do not lose this strong connection between the thumb-side of your hands and your mat as it will ground and stabilize you in the pose.

Curl your toes under, and with an exhalation, lift up into Downward-Facing Dog Pose by lifting from your abdomen and straightening your legs. Come directly onto the balls of your feet. Look at your feet and make sure two things are happening: one, your heels are slightly turned out and two, the inner and outer anklebones of each leg are parallel to each other and to the floor. In other words, be careful not to let the arches of your feet collapse downward or let the weight roll way over onto the outer border of your feet.

Inhale, and with a slow exhalation, lower your heels toward the floor with deliberate awareness, making sure they stay turned out while you're pressing them to the floor. Even if the heels do not make it all the way down, keep your intention of pressing strongly downward with the heels throughout the pose.

I often observe students practicing this pose with the hands and feet too close to each other as shown in figure 5.14. Experiment with moving your hands a few inches forward and see if there is more space for the spine to lengthen.

If this pose is easy for you, try tucking your tailbone under just a little bit to keep from over-rotating the pelvis forward and down and thus over-stretching the origin of the hamstring muscles, which are attached to the ischial tuberosities of the lower pelvis.

Now turn your attention to the shoulders. Inhale, and with the exhalation, rotate your arms internally as shown in figure 5.15.

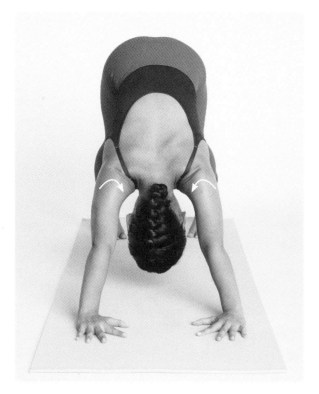

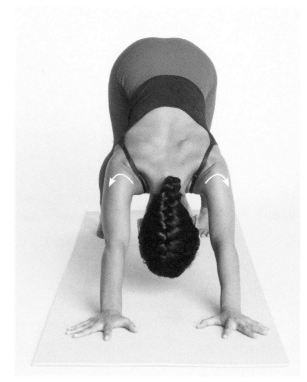

FIGURE 5.15

FIGURE 5.16

Figure 5.16 shows the model externally rotating the upper arms, which can entrap the supraspinatus tendon.

Once you have internally rotated, without lifting the little finger side of the hands, push back with your arms to create an angle of lift that is diagonal. The idea is not to press the breastbone to the floor but rather to move the energy and the body itself from the root of the hand upward and outward, so the entire vertebral column is long. Do not hang in the shoulders.

Now this is the key: let your outer shoulder blades move down and out toward your little fingers so that the scapulae are allowed and encouraged to rotate. Create a little muscular action between your shoulder blades, especially at the very lower tips, the inferior angle, as if to bring these tips slightly together. Remember to breathe as you push against the floor. Put weight on your fingers, so your wrist will feel better.

Both your upper and lower arms are internally rotating to seat the head of the humerus in the deepest aspect of the glenoid fossa, and your shoulder blades are moving *toward your head*. It might help to turn your fingertips inward a little bit. The shoulder blades actually move in one direction and the spine in the other, toward your pelvis.

Let your head hang down, and hold the pose for several breaths. Then bend your knees and, if possible, sit back on your heels with your head on the floor to rest for a moment before repeating the pose one more time.

Plank Pose

CHATURANGA DANDASANA 1

Most of this chapter has been focused on how to move from the shoulder blades in the most natural way possible when using your arms. But we need to hold the shoulder blades still, or almost still, in poses that require more stability for the whole upper extremity.

In chapter 1 we discussed the effect of gravity on the vertebral column. Gravity always shapes which muscles are working in our body and for what purpose. In Plank Pose, we are holding the entire body up horizontally against the force of gravity. This is a challenging task, and we need the shoulder joints to be as stable as possible in order to accomplish it. In Downward-Facing Dog Pose, on the other hand, we are moving more *with* the force of gravity as we let gravity pull the upper body toward the floor.

What we need from the shoulder joints in Plank Pose is to be stable, so the arms can hold us up. This means that the shoulder blades do *not rotate*, and we don't move the shoulder joint into more than 90° of flexion.

Step onto your mat and get down on your hands and the balls of your feet with your arms at 90° of flexion. Keep your breath soft and *tuck your tailbone*, drawing it under and lifting your belly button up. Remember in chapter 1 when I specifically instructed not to tuck? That was because you were in a completely different relationship to gravity than you are now. You were vertical, standing in Mountain Pose.

In this pose, however, we need to recruit the abdominal muscles to contract powerfully to hold the rib cage and the pelvis together against the strong force of gravity that is acting to pull your body downward toward the floor.

Lift your thoracic spine (mid-back) higher than your shoulder blades, so you are slightly flexing or rounding your upper back. Do not allow the mid-back to sag down or arch below the level of the shoulder blades. When you are sagging, you are literally hanging on your shoulder capsule and not using muscles to maintain the pose. Your shoulder joints will be much more stable and effective to help you practice the pose when you lift up with the thoracic spine.

Additionally, it is quite important that your hands and arms are exactly underneath your shoulder joints. This absolute vertical line between the center of the shoulder joint and the center of the wrist joint creates a more congruent relationship in the glenohumeral joint. In other words, this position of the arms creates a very stable relationship between the head of your humerus and the receiving concavity of the glenoid fossa. The more

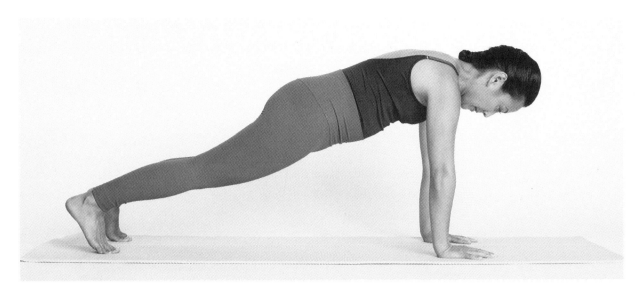

FIGURE 5.17

congruence here, the more stable the joint. Thus, stability in the shoulder joint in Plank Pose comes first from the position of the scapula and secondarily from the verticality of the arms.

Keep your head in line with the rest of your body, and breathe a few breaths. Come back down to your hands and knees, rest a bit, and then repeat the pose.

Four-Legged Staff Pose

CHATURANGA DANDASANA 2

Start in Plank Pose and then bend your elbows to come down toward the floor. Make sure your shoulder blades are moving toward your waist.

Keep your elbows at a natural distance from your body. You do not need to grip them in, but don't let them fly out either. Think of moving the back of your upper arms toward the elbows; imagine the elbows themselves are pressing down toward the floor.

If you allow the shoulder blades to move toward your ears, you will destabilize your shoulder joints and make the pose much harder. Always remember that the shoulder blades in Four-Legged Staff Pose are moving down your back and slightly together.

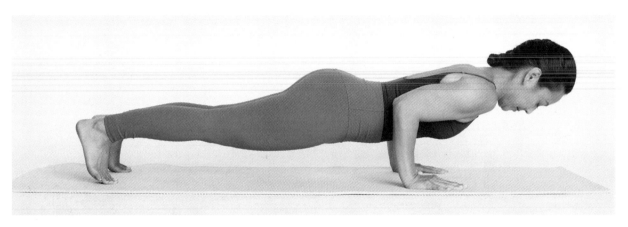

FIGURE 5.18

Be sure to lift your belly up by using your abdominal muscles. Sometimes it helps to squeeze your legs tightly toward one another; this action recruits help from the strong leg muscles like the adductors of the inner thigh, and this can really help to hold you up. Remember to breathe even though you are very active.

Imagine your hands pushing you backward on the floor while your toes are pushing you forward at the same time. This will give you the sensation of lifting up in the center of your body. Come down before you are overly tired. Rest and repeat one or two more times.

Caution: if you have osteoporosis or any problem with the integrity of your ribs, do not practice the variation with the belt that follows.

If you are struggling with this pose, you are not alone. Try using your belt. Sit on the floor and fasten the belt in a circle. Slip the belt on your arms so it is just above your elbows. The bottom border of the belt is at the end of your upper arm, just where the bend of the elbow joint starts.

The belt should be loose enough to allow your elbows to move toward the side of your body. Do not make the belt so tight that it interferes with this ability or with the positioning of the shoulder blades described above.

Now take the pose. Keep breathing. Position yourself so that the belt is holding your body on your bottom ribs. The belt will now act like a "sling" to help hold your body up. Let the weight of your body be on your hands, feet, and the belt.

Now that the pose will likely seem much easier, you can spend some time noticing the position of your shoulder blades, elbows, and hands. The belt is a great help to those new to the pose, so if you are a teacher, you will have time to instruct students in the technique of the pose without the fear of them overdoing it. They can also be more relaxed in the pose.

As before, draw your shoulder blades down and also drop your elbows. Do not choose a hand position that is too far back from directly under your shoulder joints or that is too much in front of them. Observe the model's hand position. Generally, the hand needs to be well under the shoulder because that is where the body actually needs the support and lift.

Hold the position on the belt for several breaths before coming down by lying down, bending your knees, and using your arms to come to a hands-and-knees position, and then sit back. Rest, and then try again.

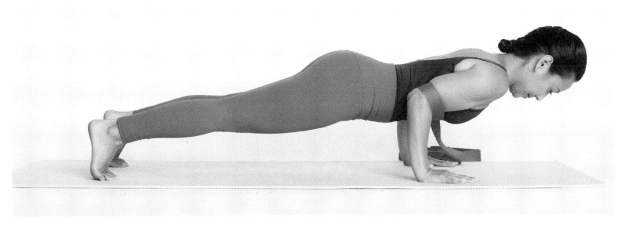

FIGURE 5.19

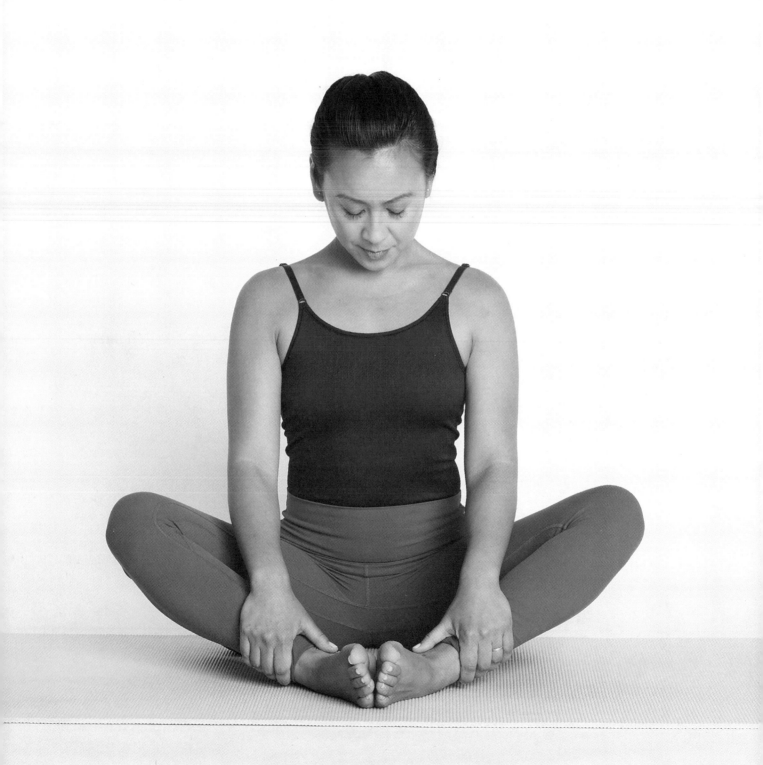

6

Aligning the Knees

YOUR KNEES ARE MORE COMPLICATED THAN YOU THINK

We are as young as our knees.

Y EARS AGO, I was taking a class in a completely different system of yoga asana than I was accustomed to practicing. The teacher was famous and very adamant that we do exactly what he said to do.

Midway through the class, he told us to practice a pose in which we began by sitting on the floor in an easy cross-legged position. He began to instruct Root Lock Pose (Mulabandhasana). We were to take one foot and bring it close to the groin, then turn the toes down and the heel forward and up, and finally turn the toes completely backward so that our toes were pointing toward the wall behind us and the arch of the foot was on the ground. The final instruction was to sit on that foot. I am not making this up. This pose obviously required a tremendous amount of laxity in the structures of the inner knee, to say the least.

I had never attempted such an action, and I learned immediately and convincingly that my knees simply do not do that. I made an honest attempt at this pose, and then I wisely backed off when met with pain. Nevertheless, I was summarily scolded by the teacher and told I was being too lazy.

Although I was young and very flexible, I did not have a knee joint that would allow me to do this pose. To this day I am so grateful that I did not let that teacher, or my ego, cause me to force my knees to do what they simply could not structurally do.

My hope for you is that with the help of this chapter, you will not only learn about how your knees work and how to keep them safe, but you will also learn to trust what your knees are "telling" you during your practice of asana.

Why You Need to Know This

The knee is arguably the most complicated joint to be found in the human body. While the shoulder joints are complicated too, the knees have the additional challenge of being weight-bearing joints; the shoulder joints rarely are.

The main reason for this complication is that the knee is the "prisoner" of the hip joint and the foot. The knee is subject to all sorts of impact, shear, and torsion forces that act on it because it is in the middle of the kinetic (movement) chain bounded by the hip and foot/ankle.

Yoga asana require a lot from the knees. We stretch all the supporting structures in front of, behind, and on the sides of the knee. We bend and twist them, use them to do Lotus Pose (Padmasana), kneel on them, and compress them deeply in Child's Pose (Balasana). Unfortunately, we often take our knees for granted. Remember how easy it was for you as a teenager to run up the stairs two at a time? Not so easy for many of us to do this after we've accumulated some life mileage. Like the rest of our body, the knees age, and this fact needs to be acknowledged and allowed for *even if there is no pain in our knees* when we are practicing on our own or taking a class.

The knees are susceptible to strain injuries in part because, unlike the hip joint, the knee joint does not have the same amount of bulky muscular support. Look at all the muscles around your hip joint that help keep it stable. You will see lots of huge muscles, and the hip joint itself is deep and designed for stability and also for movement in many different directions.

The knees are different. For one thing, the knee joint surfaces are much shallower and therefore less stable joints than the hips. The muscles around the knee are nowhere near as large or as powerful as those at the hip joint. And, thanks to their position in the kinetic chain of the legs, the knees undergo some intense forces as we move. These forces, coupled with a knee alignment that is not perfect, can contribute mightily to deterioration in knee cartilage and place stress on the soft tissues like ligaments and tendons that surround the joint. Additionally, research has found that every pound of body weight we have is translated directly into four pounds of weight onto the knee joint itself. Multiply those four pounds by gravity plus impact, and we have an equation for wear and tear.

The medial, or inner knee, has a unique relationship with some of the muscles around it, which makes what happens to the muscles outside the joint directly affect what happens to the interior knee joint. This is not true for the outer, or lateral, knee joint.

For these reasons, and others, it is easy to see why we need to understand our knees and treat them with deep respect and maybe even with admiration for all they allow us to do. Spend some time taking in the anatomy facts and illustrations in the next section. Hopefully they will help you understand your knees and give them the appreciation and care they deserve.

Your Structure

The knee joint proper is created by the union of the femur and the tibia. The fibula, on the lateral side of the lower leg, is not directly part of the knee joint. However, it acts as a strut to give stability to the knee, the lateral leg, the ankle, and the foot.

The patella (kneecap), which forms during the first year of life, is the "roof" of the knee joint and rests in the tendon of the quadriceps muscle. The patella has two main functions. One is to protect the anterior joint from injury. The patella allows us to kneel. We even have a special fat pad and fluid-filled sacs called bursae to make kneeling more comfortable.

The other main purpose of the patella is to function as a lever so that the power of the quadriceps muscle in knee extension is multiplied when we need to straighten our knee, especially if force is needed, like when we are kicking a ball. Because the tendon of the quadriceps travels up and over the patella as it moves down to where it joins the upper tibia, the force of the muscle in contraction is increased. The slight elevation provided by the patella is like a fulcrum for the tendon of the quadriceps muscle where it attaches to the patella. This slight elevation is quite effective in increasing the power of the contractions of the quadriceps into a more efficient and powerful extensor force to straighten the knee joint.

You may have heard of the two important ligaments in your knee called the cruciate ligaments. The word *cruciate* means "cross-shaped." The cruciate

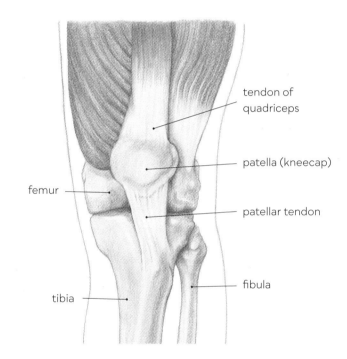

FIGURE 6.1
Anterior view of the left knee

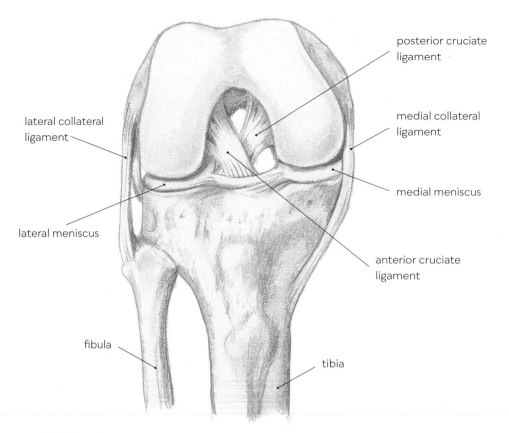

FIGURE 6.2
Anterior view of right knee

ligaments, like all ligaments, hold bones to bones and actually make an X shape inside the knee joint, thus their name.

The anterior cruciate ligament (ACL) and the posterior cruciate ligament (PCL) are named for where they originate, which is on the anterior or posterior tibia. They function to disallow excessive movement in the knee joint, especially in flexion and extension.

The ACL, typically the more likely of the two to be injured, prevents hyperextension of the knee joint. Hyperextension of the knee means that the knee joint is able to straighten past a vertical line when standing. In standing, a person with hyperextended knees will appear to have a tibia that is positioned backward, past the vertical line. You can observe this in many yoga students if you look at them from the side in Mountain Pose.

When we habitually stand with the pelvis pushed well forward, one of the compensations the body makes is to hyperextend the knee joints. This action, of course, is made to help us adapt to the ubiquitous force of gravity. If you, or one of your students, has hyperextended knees, take care not to practice yoga asana in a manner that makes this worse.

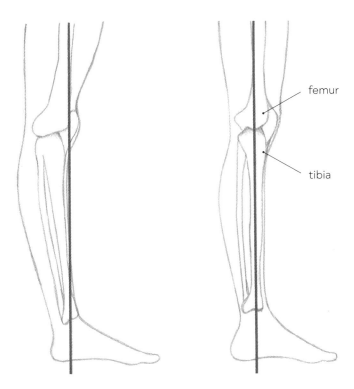

femur

tibia

hyperextended knee joint

normal alignment knee joint showing maximal congruence between the femur and tibia

FIGURE 6.3

I believe that hyperextension can be created by poor postural habits in childhood and youth. Being born with naturally loose ligaments may also be a cause. The main problem with having hyperextended knees is that such a knee is less stable than one that has a normal range of extension. This means that when completely straight, the knee joint is in a straight line. In a hyperextended knee, there is too much movement allowed, the tibia pushes back past the vertical line, and this puts strain on other tissues in the knee and around it.

Here is a simple way to see if you have hyperextended knees. Sit on the floor in Staff Pose (Dandasana) with your spine long and your legs together and stretched straight out in front of you. Now roll your thighbones to a neutral position so the kneecaps are looking at the ceiling. Strongly contract your quadriceps (upper thigh) muscles. Notice the tendency to stretch out through your heels. Resist this urge; keep your feet completely and totally relaxed, practically floppy.

If your feet are relaxed, not pulled up toward you, and yet your heels lift off the floor, you have hyperextended knees. If you can contract your quadriceps strongly, keep your feet completely relaxed, and your heels do not lift no matter how hard you contract your quadriceps, then you likely don't have hyperextended knees.

If you have hyperextended knees, avoid squatting for long periods of time in yoga asana practice. The ACL is very stretched in a squatting position. However, the most stress on the ACL is at both 30° and 90° of flexion when bearing weight. This means that standing poses where your knee is flexed at a 90° angle, like Extended Side Angle Pose (please review chapter 3, page 50), hold the increased potential for stress and injury to the ACL; be sure to practice these types of poses with pristine alignment.

The PCL prevents the anterior and posterior (front to back and back to front) movements of the tibia on the femur and the femur on the tibia. The PCL is injured when the tibia is forced suddenly and traumatically backward, like in an auto accident when the knee jams into the dashboard, and the tibia is strongly moved backward. Injuries to the PCL are definitely rarer in yoga than injuries to the ACL.

But by far, the medial knee is the most vulnerable part of the knee joint and is thus susceptible to injury. This is true in part because structures located outside the knee joint proper can, and do, directly affect the health of the structures inside of the knee joint. This is not true for the anatomy of the lateral knee joint.

One such structure that is outside of the knee joint and yet can affect it internally is the tendinous attachment of the semimembranosus muscle, one of the medial hamstring muscles. Remember that tendons join muscles to bones. The semimembranosus originates at the ischial tuberosity of the pelvis and is attached in part to the medial collateral ligament on the inside of the knee joint. (This ligament will be discussed in more detail below.)

When we stretch this muscle, and thus its tendinous attachment, in standing poses, forward bends, and also sometimes when we are sitting in Wide-Angle Seated Forward Bend, we need to be aware of the inner knee. Be especially aware that you do not allow too much stretch to be created in the semimembranosus muscle where it attaches at the inner knee. If you do, you could be adversely affecting your medial collateral ligament as well, which is found deeper in the structure of the knee joint.

Never forget that if you have pain in or around a joint where the muscles attach to the bone, this is not a healthy

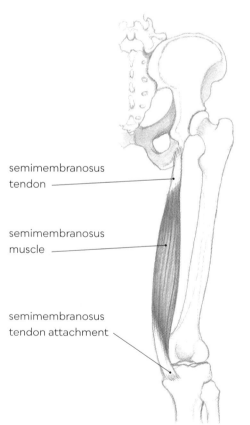

semimembranosus tendon

semimembranosus muscle

semimembranosus tendon attachment

FIGURE 6.4

pain. If you feel pain in the knee joint, or any joint for that matter, stop what you are doing and pay attention. You may want to seek out advice from your health-care professional about this type of pain. Healthy yoga asana stretches are to be felt in the belly of the muscle or in the fascial tissue that is in or covering a muscle, not near or in a joint.

Another knee structure deeper in the knee joint that has connection with a more exterior structure is the medial cartilage, or meniscus. There are actually two separate cartilages in the knee joint. One is on the medial or inner side and is the larger of the two. The other one is to be found on the lateral or outer side.

The medial meniscus, as well as the lateral one, functions to create space between the end of the femur and top of the tibia. This space allows room for normal movements of the knee joint. In several ways, the menisci are akin in structure and function to the intervertebral discs of the vertebral column.

The meniscus adds padding between the bones. Because the meniscus has a deep, thick, ring-like shape, it also serves to increase the depth of the joint surface where the tibia and femur meet, thus contributing to stability in the joint as well by creating a deeper articular (joint) surface.

The medial meniscus attaches to a ligament mentioned earlier: the medial collateral ligament. This ligament, sometimes called the tibial collateral ligament, holds the medial tibia and femur together at the inner knee, thus giving stability to your medial knee joint. The medial collateral ligament also resists twisting movements. The lateral collateral ligament connects the fibula to the femur and creates stability on the outer side of the knee.

At the inner knee, the medial collateral ligament connects directly to the medial meniscus located inside the knee joint. Again, remember that whatever affects your inner knee on the outside of your joint can affect your interior medial knee structures, like the medial cartilage. If you overstretch your medial collateral ligament, you could damage your medial meniscus or, at the very least, create the potential for damage.

Because of the tissue connections around the medial knee, this is the place where so many knee injuries occur. The knee injuries that come from yoga are usually not sudden; they are often slow to show themselves. It is like water dripping on a stone. Drop by drop the water will wear a hole in the stone, even though it has taken years or centuries to do so.

I believe that many knee injuries in yoga asana practice are created by a similar process: practicing in a manner that is a little out of alignment, with a little too much stress on the knee joint. Over time, the knee pays the cost. Let's learn new ways of using our knees in asana practice that do not harm them.

Your Anatomy in Action

Though it is a commonly held belief, the knee is *not* a hinge joint only. When we bend and straighten it, the knee joint moves in three ways: it rolls, glides, and rotates in a perfect choreography that is fascinating to observe. Understanding these movements in three dimensions is beyond the scope of this book. However, it is important to remember that our knee movements are sophisticated and that they often depend on their relationship to the foot on the floor. When the foot is fixed to the floor, like it is when you are standing up from a chair, this relationship is called a closed kinetic chain.

Knee movements are subtly different when the foot is not fixed to the floor, as when you lie on your back on your yoga mat and then bend your knee to your chest. The foot is not connected to the floor; it is free. This is termed an open kinetic chain.

The most important point here is to begin to observe what your knee is doing in poses and never to push it to move into an extreme position just because you can. I hope we can learn to practice yoga asana with respect for this astounding joint that serves us all day with a great deal of movement intelligence.

One way we can begin to get to know our own knee joints better is by improving our power of observation. It is possible to see and feel fairly easily one of the three movements that occur in the knee joint: rotation. Begin your observation now by trying this.

Stand on your yoga mat and prepare for Extended Side Angle Pose. For directions on practicing this pose, please review chapter 3, page 50). You only will need to attempt the very first part of the pose in order to feel rotation in the knee.

Stand with your feet in position for the pose with your legs wide apart. You should have your right foot turned out a little more than 90° and your left, or back foot, turned inward about 45°. Now put your attention on your right tibia, specifically the bony protuberance front and center on your tibia. This anatomical landmark is called the tibial tuberosity.

Inhale, and as you exhale, bend your right knee over your little toe as you begin to move into the pose. Do this slowly. Note the position of your tibia as well as the relationship between your patella and your tibial tuberosity. Try this several times and you will begin to feel the rotation that is happening from your knee joint.

This is a normal movement for the joint. When the thigh is fixed, the tibia can rotate; when the foot and leg are fixed, the thigh can rotate. This is

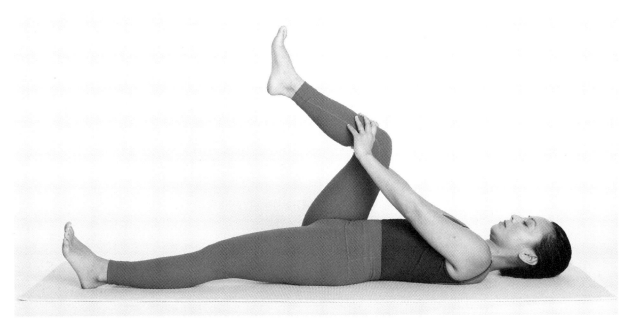

FIGURE 6.5

what happens to the knee joint in flexion, and it is easier to feel in a closed kinetic chain.

Try bending your knee again, and this time hold your thigh with your hand firmly enough to feel this external rotation of the thigh, but not so firmly as to interfere with this natural process.

Once you have felt this external rotation, bend your knee once more and pay attention to the relationship between your femur and tibia as you slowly straighten your knee. You may observe and/or feel your femur rotate internally as you slowly straighten your knee. Try it several times. Be sure to keep your knee pointing almost even behind your foot, a bit toward your little toe. Do not let your femur drop inward, so it is in line with the big toe side of your foot. If you do this, you will stress the knee joint, even if you don't feel it.

As you straighten your knee, you will begin to notice that the tibia rotates internally on the stable femur. Again, this is normal movement for your knee joint in a closed kinetic chain when you straighten your knee against gravity.

These movements are normal when the foot is fixed to the floor and are part of the way the knee creates flexion (bending) and extension (straightening). Don't forget that the surfaces in the knee are also rolling and gliding during these flexion and extension movements.

To feel this rotation in an open kinetic chain, lie on your back on your yoga mat. With an exhalation, raise one straight leg up toward you. Now put your hands around your upper tibia; hold it firmly enough to feel it well into your hands but lightly enough to allow it to move naturally.

Keeping your hands around your upper calf, slowly bend your knee. (See figure 6.5.) While it won't be as dramatic as the external and internal rotation that you felt and saw in standing, it is still possible to feel the external rotation. This is the tibia rotating internally on the femur in an open kinetic chain.

As you straighten your knee with your hands around your calf, feel the external rotation of the tibia. Repeat bending and straightening your knee with your hands in place several times in succession. Rotation of the tibia should clearly be happening.

I think it is important to try these two attempts at feeling and understanding what happens to your knee joint in movement. Then it will become more apparent that the knee moves in a much more sophisticated way than just with the action of a hinge. When you straighten your knee in an open kinetic chain, there is also external rotation of the tibia, but it is not as easy to feel with your hands.

In an open kinetic chain, the tibia internally rotates on flexion and externally rotates on extension. In a closed kinetic chain, like a standing pose, the femur externally rotates on flexion, and internally rotates on extension. This is normal and desirable and is called the screw home mechanism.

Thus when we bend the knee to begin Extended Side Angle Pose, for example, the femur naturally externally rotates. When we straighten to come out of the pose, the femur naturally internally rotates.

These passive, rotational joint movements that accompany extension and flexion help to make the knee more stable by bringing the tibia and the femur into their neutral positions for a more secure weight-bearing position in the joint. This position of the knee in full extension will be discussed further in the "Attentive Practice" section of this chapter when we discuss knee position in Mountain Pose and Downward-Facing Dog Pose.

In standing, walking, and practicing yoga asana, the knee joint is always balancing stability and mobility. The most stable position for the knee joint is extension, with standing extension being more stable than sitting extension. The most mobile position is flexion, with standing flexion being more mobile than sitting flexion.

Yoga asana that are done by bending the knee in standing, i.e., weight-bearing, are the asana in which the knee is the most vulnerable to misuse and injury. One reason is that when you bend your knee to a 90° angle like we sometimes do in

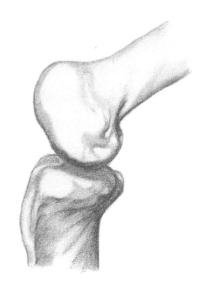

FIGURE 6.6
Knee flexion showing reduced congruence and reduced stability in the joint during standing

standing poses, you have greatly reduced the congruence between the femur and the tibia. The less congruence in the joint surfaces, the less stable the knee joint will be.

Not only do we practice poses in which the knee is bearing weight while being in a position of lesser stability, we also actually hold these positions against the force of gravity with lots of our weight on the flexed joint.

I am not suggesting that we stop practicing these types of poses; rather, I am suggesting that when we do, we make a specific choice. That choice is to make it our priority to focus on alignment and stability before range of movement. When we focus on the alignment of the feet, legs, and pelvis in Extended Side Angle Pose, for example, we may not go as far down into the pose, but by meticulously aligning our bones in the pose without striving to maximize our range of movement, we are so much less likely to get hurt.

Let the range of movement come slowly over time and focus on cultivating stability through alignment from the beginning. Do not sacrifice alignment for the sake of wanting to put your hand on the floor or in some other way prove that you have completed the pose and are a more "advanced" student. If you practice first with alignment in mind, then range, your knees will thank you. I like to say, "Choose alignment first, and the range of movement will gradually choose you."

Another important anatomical fact to remember in order to keep your knees safe in asana practice is that the knee is always the prisoner of the hip and the foot. This means that you cannot move your knee independently of the hip and the foot. This may seem obvious, but sadly it often isn't. Try to rotate your knee externally in standing without affecting your hip joint. The knee must also respond to the position of the foot. When you fix your foot to the floor, knee movements are limited by foot position. Pay attention to this anatomical fact, and your knees will be happier.

As stated previously, the knee is always balancing stability and mobility. Some yoga positions do not challenge the knee's flexibility, but rather its stability, but probably not in the way you might imagine.

Two poses that challenge the stability of the knee are the standing poses Warrior III (Virabhadrasana III) and Half Moon Pose (Ardha Chandrasana). Both of these require the student to be balanced on one leg. Both are poses in which the body is horizontal and there is the tremendous downward force of gravity to be reckoned with all along the body.

Many students mistakenly, and no doubt unconsciously, attempt to create more stability in the standing/supporting knee by pushing backward on the knee, perhaps into some degree of hyperextension. However, this position of the leg is actually less stable, and what would remedy the situation is a perfect alignment and congruence at the knee joint. In other words, the knee needs to be positioned at 0°, meaning perfectly straight, to maximize stability between the femur and the tibia.

Here is an experiment with stability that you can try in these two poses. Take your mat near a wall in case you choose to use it for balance. Stand three feet or so away from the wall, and bend forward at the same time as you lift your straight right leg backward so that your trunk and your right leg are parallel to the floor. Touch the wall with your fingertips if you wish. When you are in the full pose, slightly bend your supporting left knee to approximately 30°. This causes more muscle activity to happen. It is perhaps counterintuitive, but by creating more instability, you "wake up" the muscles that need to be active to maintain you in the pose.

Keep your breath soft, and moving gently and with great attention begin to straighten you knee. But do this with the very careful awareness of pulling all the muscles of your leg upward. Imagine the "pulling up" you do with your socks when you put them on and apply that image to your leg muscles: they all move up.

This image may contribute to creating muscle actions that will help you to feel more stable in the pose. Perhaps this way of working in these poses will prevent hyperextension or, at least, prevent you from pushing back on the knee into the direction of hyperextension.

Attentive Practice

Healthy knees are critical to our asana practice and our life. We were meant to move. Pay attention to how your movements in this section affect your knees.

CAUTIONS

Be cautious with your knees when practicing these poses, especially if you already have pain in your knee joints. This type of pain is not a healthy pain. If a movement causes discomfort in a joint, you may want to consider a consultation with your health-care provider before continuing.

PROPS NEEDED

- Nonslip yoga mat
- Full-length mirror
- Bolster
- Yoga blanket

Mountain Pose
TADASANA

Place your mat facing a full-length mirror, and begin with Tadasana. This pose always begins with the feet. Stand with the outside of your feet exactly parallel to the edges of your mat and with the normal curves in your vertebral column, especially the lumbosacral spine. Make sure your knees are exposed and notice the placement of your kneecaps.

Normal kneecaps face slightly medially, or inward. They do not face straight ahead. That is a yoga myth. The reason your kneecaps face inward is because of the nature of the relationship between the head of the femur and the hip socket. The head of the femur sits in the hip joint at an angle so that the trochanter is actually in front of the acetabulum as was discussed in chapter 3 (see figure 3.4). This is the neutral position of the hip joint.

Stand in front of the mirror in Mountain Pose (see chapter 1, page 11 for instructions on this pose). Make sure that the outside border of your feet, the little toe side, is exactly parallel to the edge of your yoga mat. While this alignment works for most students, you may find it more comfortable to position your feet so that the space between your second and third toe is oriented directly forward. This position may also help you avoid overpronating (flattening) your feet. Usually students turn their feet out in Mountain Pose, which ensures that the hip joint will not be in neutral and that the kneecaps are pointing outward.

Now look at your kneecaps in the mirror. Are they pointing inward? Outward? Do they look symmetrical? Sometimes one points slightly in and the other points forward or even laterally. All combinations of placement are possible.

If you notice a discrepancy, and/or if you have knee pain or dysfunction, my suggestion is that you seek out the help of a physical therapist who specializes in manual therapy or an experienced bodyworker, perhaps, who is well trained in the technique of myofascial release, the work of physical therapist John Barnes.

The neutral and desirable position of the kneecaps is that they face slightly inward. If this is not the position of your kneecaps, the probable reason could be a muscle imbalance in your thigh muscles and/or soft tissue imbalances in the muscles surrounding your hip joints or other surrounding tissues.

It is important to address this imbalance so that your kneecaps can track evenly, healthily, and smoothly over the joint with the femur. The better the alignment of your kneecaps, the less wear and tear you put on the joint between kneecap and femur, and that promotes a lifetime of healthy movement in your knees.

Downward-Facing Dog Pose

ADHO MUKHA SVANASANA

Downward-Facing Dog Pose was taught previously in chapter 5 on pages 86–87, so please check those pictures. The emphasis there was on the healthy action in the glenohumeral joints in the shoulders, as well as on the free movement of the scapulae, which creates the full shoulder flexion required in order for this pose to be pain free and enjoyable. In this chapter, we will focus on the position of the knee joints in Downward-Facing Dog Pose.

Before you practice Downward-Facing Dog Pose, look at figure 6.7.

This is a drawing showing the positioning of the kneecaps and the femur in a neutral position. If the drawing showed the kneecaps facing straight ahead, that would actually mean the femurs were externally rotated. If the kneecaps in the drawing were facing medially (inward) more than they are, that would mean the femurs were internally rotated. Remember that the neutral kneecap position when the knee is fully extended like it is in Mountain Pose and Downward-Facing Dog Pose is slightly medially placed.

Step onto your mat and take the Downward-Facing Dog Pose. Make sure your feet and hands are far enough apart from each other that your spine can stretch up and out in a diagonal direction past and above your pelvis, and that it is not forced to sag or drop down. Release your neck and let your head hang down. Keep the breath soft.

Now look at your kneecaps. They should be facing slightly inward as explained above. Try turning your heels slightly out to stretch your inner calf and to help internally rotate your thighs. The inner calf muscle is much larger than the outer muscle, and for most people, it typically needs more stretching. The outer head of the gastrocnemius—the superficial calf muscle on the lateral proximal side—also helps to flex the knee, so it needs to be stretched with the hamstrings that are knee flexors as well.

Spend some time making changes in the position of your feet and in the rotation of your thighs so that the kneecaps are turning slightly medially. If this does not happen, ask for help from your yoga teacher and/or seek out a professional bodyworker to help you create a more aligned kneecap position.

Hold the pose for a few breaths and notice how your foot and thigh position affects the position of your kneecaps. Come down, and repeat one more time.

Teachers: When you look at the backs of your student's knees, there should be a diagonal line at the bottom of the back of the knee that points downward from the back outer knee toward the inner knee. If that line is more horizontal, they are not turning the femurs and/or tibias internally, and the tibias and kneecaps might be moving too much in a lateral direction.

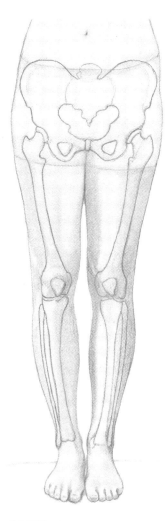

FIGURE 6.7
Anterior knee joint showing normal slight internal rotation of patella (kneecaps) in Mountain Pose

Lotus Pose

PADMASANA

This is one of the most challenging asana for many people. It should be approached with deep respect and care. The first question to ask yourself is this: To Lotus or not to Lotus? How do you know if you are ready for Lotus Pose? How can you tell if you will be able to attempt the pose with a reasonable assurance that it will be safe?

Here is what I suggest. Sit on the floor with the soles of your feet together in Bound Angle Pose (Baddha Konasana) as shown in figure 6.8. Place your feet approximately six to eight inches away from your body.

Take note of two things. First, are you able to roll your pubic bones forward and down so that you are sitting in front of your sitting bones? Is your pelvis able to tip forward easily, or do you feel that you are rolling backward and are stuck there? Is your chest sinking because your lumbar and thoracic spine are flexed, and your thoracic curve is increased because of your pelvic position?

To be safe, it is imperative that you can roll your pelvis forward, press the pubic bone toward the floor, and maintain normal curves in your back. If this is the case, then take note of the second factor. How high are your knees from the floor? To proceed with Lotus Pose, it is best if your knees are below the rim of your pelvis and almost on the floor. If not, do not try full Lotus Pose.

If you are ready to proceed, pick up your right lower leg by scooping your hands underneath your calf, with your right hand deeply into the back of the knee joint and your left hand at about midcalf level or a little lower. With your left hand, rotate the flesh of your calf outward and down.

Stretch out strongly with your heel as you bring your toes toward your shinbone so that the outer and inner ankles are straight from side to side. Do not sickle or curve your foot by pulling on it. In fact, do not pull on your foot at all to come into Lotus Pose. If you practice the pose with a sickled ankle, you will put a lot of stress on the outer ankle ligaments. Additionally, you can stress the gap between your lateral knee

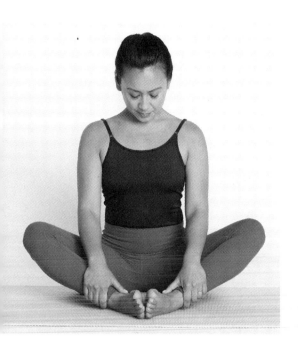

FIGURE 6.8

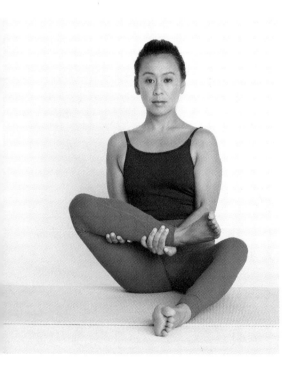

FIGURE 6.9

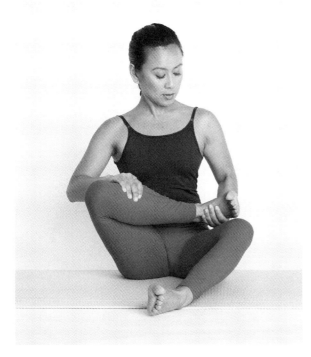

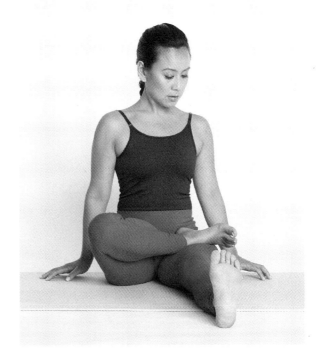

FIGURE 6.10

FIGURE 6.11

structures, overstretch ligaments around the fibular head, and put more pressure on your medial knee compartment. Not a good idea.

These ligaments are the ones most likely to be injured in an ankle sprain, and you want these ligaments to have a lot of integrity so that your ankle remains stable, on the mat and off. Once stretched, the lateral ankle ligaments may heal, but they are more susceptible to further injury.

It is very important that you are meticulous about turning your right calf flesh slightly outward and upward and your tibia out and down as you prepare to place your foot on your other leg. Remember that open chain knee flexion is accompanied by an internal rotation of the tibia; balance this rotation as you come into Lotus Pose, and you will be helping your body do what it naturally does. I think this specific technique can be protective of your knees.

With the right lower leg lifted, stretch out through your heel, and reach under and hold your outside right ankle with your left palm up, but keep your right palm down as you turn your right upper calf muscles outward and down away from you.

Now use your left hand to guide your right heel high up on your left thigh. Keep stretching out strongly with your right heel until the foot is actually resting on your thigh. Try to place your right heel just inside your left ASIS (hip bone).

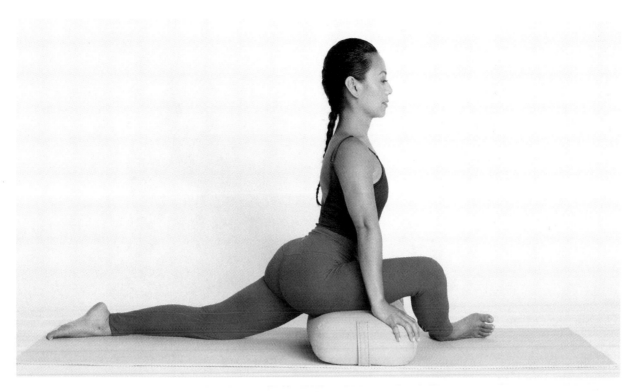

FIGURE 6.12

Once the foot is placed and you let go with your hands, relax the foot. It will slightly curve upward, but that should be minimal. The weight of the lower leg is on the left thigh, so that the upper thigh is bearing the weight of the lower leg and not the foot. Do not place only the foot on the left thigh, but a portion of your lower leg so that the foot is almost free.

If this is impossible for you now, do not force the pose; instead continue working on increasing the flexibility of the external rotator muscles of your hip with a stretch like the one shown in figure 6.12.

In this stretch, notice how the model is putting most of the weight of her right leg on her left top thigh. Her right tibia is parallel to the edge of her mat, and she is twisting toward the front leg by exhaling and moving her belly toward the leg. Use your breathing, moving on exhalation.

You can also use greater height under your pelvis if you need it. Your hands can support you while you sit upright, or like the model, you can lean forward or even come down onto your forearms and then walk toward the right. This will be a strong stretch for most people. Whichever arm position you choose, it is important to keep the weight on the left side of the body and internally rotate your left leg. That means your toes will point inward, toward the right.

Make sure that if you practice this hip rotator pose, that your front tibia is exactly parallel to the short end of your mat, and that your front heel is exactly in line with the middle of your knee. Additionally, your back leg should be strongly internally rotating, so that your kneecap faces toward the right and does not turn out externally. This brings your weight onto your top back thigh. Imagine that you are pushing downward from your top outer back thigh as you rotate.

Be sure to use a bolster even if your "hips are open" to protect your front knee. You can add a blanket to the bolster to increase the height. The stretch should be strong but pleasant on your outer side hip.

You can aid the process of completing Lotus Pose by lifting your right hip up a little bit from the floor and moving it forward with your leg as you place your lower leg on your opposite thigh. This technique of moving your lower leg by moving your pelvis and your hip joint together with the leg will make your Lotus Pose surprisingly more comfortable.

Now comes an important moment. Begin the whole process of bringing your left leg into Lotus Pose. Move

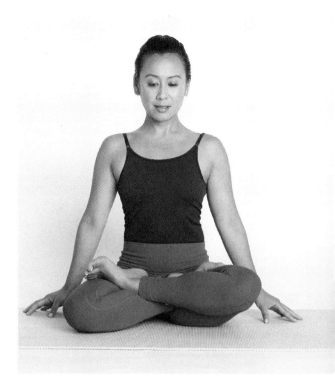

FIGURE 6.13

even more meticulously than you did before. Be sure to rotate the tibia down and out and the calf flesh up and out as you begin to place your left leg. But equally important is to press the head of your left femur downward and thus enhance the external rotation of the hip joint as you do this.

Very slowly begin to pass your left lower leg over your right lower leg. This should be fairly easy to do. Under no circumstances force the left leg on top of the right. Remember the tip of moving from the hip, actually taking the weight off your left buttock a bit so you can move your left hip socket forward and then place the leg.

Sit in Lotus Pose for five to ten breaths, then slowly help your left leg to come out, then your right. You may want to stand up and walk around for a few steps before trying the other side.

Do not be surprised if Lotus Pose to the other side feels quite different than the first side. If you continue practicing this pose, always move into the pose slowly and with respect, even if the pose feels easy for you. And always practice both sides.

In my practice I alternate legs: one week I work mostly on bringing the right leg in first; the next week I work mostly on the left leg first. Sometimes I try to sit in one side during the first part of teaching Deep Relaxation Pose in my classes. After many years of practicing in this way, I sometimes forget which leg is my favorite to bring in first.

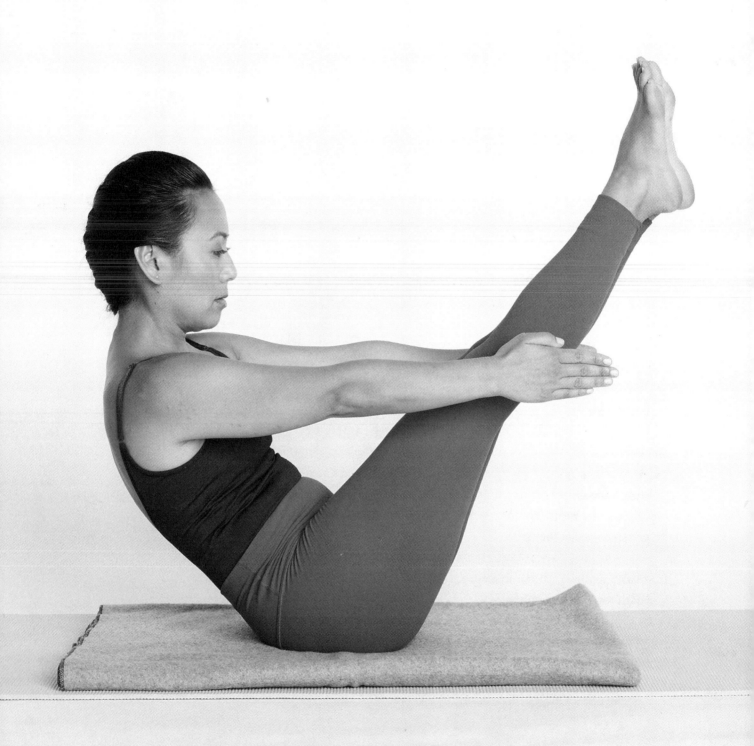

7

Skip the Sit-Ups

IT'S ALL ABOUT STABILIZATION

We all have a "six pack." You just can't see it on some of us.

W HEN I SAW my first yoga teacher demonstrate Boat Pose (Navasana), I thought it looked so easy. Then I tried it. I struggled more than I thought I would. My top thighs were burning, and my lower back was complaining. I tried harder, but it just made it worse, and I really did not feel much contraction in my "abs" at all as I was instructed to do.

When I began to study anatomy seriously, I became better acquainted with the fascinating abdominal muscles. They are arranged in layers and create an interesting pattern on the front and sides of the trunk. Like everyone else, I believed that sit-ups were the best thing to do to create a strong abdomen, and I diligently did many sit-ups, but it didn't seem to help much. My Boat Pose still felt unpleasant. I chalked it up to weak abdominals and kept doing sit-ups.

I was eventually to learn that my approach to creating strong abdominal muscles was based on a key misunderstanding I had about the way these muscles functioned during movements. I was not living in anatomical reality when I believed and acted as if my abdominal muscles were best strengthened with sit-ups. When I corrected that misunderstanding, and then applied my new knowledge to Boat Pose, not only was the pose much easier, but I also actually began to like doing it. I want to share with you in this chapter the knowledge I have gained about how the abdominals really work.

Why You Need to Know This

In chapter 1 we discussed the effect the force of gravity has all the time on how and when our muscles work. When we incorporate this knowledge about gravity into our yoga practice, and in our daily life, it makes a big difference in our comfort and safety.

The abdominal muscles have a number of jobs. They function to support the abdominal organs and the vertebral column and to aid in forceful breathing. They also maintain the intra-abdominal pressure needed during childbirth and when coughing and defecating.

But the main function of the abdominal muscles is to stabilize the ribs and pelvis, i.e., the trunk, to hold them together if you will, against the force of gravity. This is true in sitting, standing, walking, and all the other activities of daily life. The abdominal muscles move and stabilize our trunk.

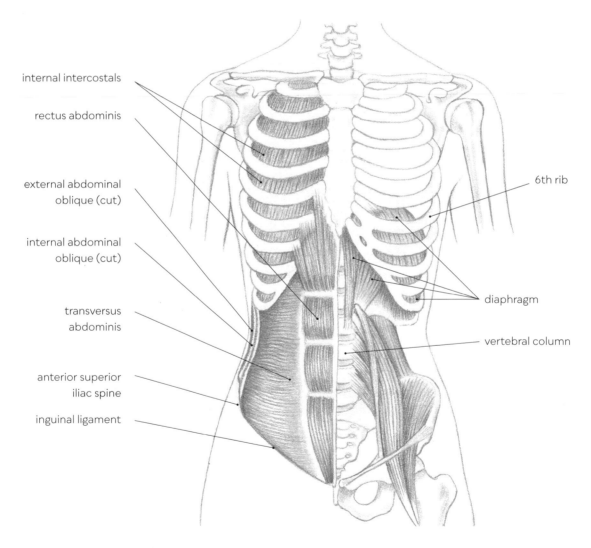

internal intercostals

rectus abdominis

external abdominal oblique (cut)

internal abdominal oblique (cut)

transversus abdominis

anterior superior iliac spine

inguinal ligament

6th rib

diaphragm

vertebral column

FIGURE 7.1
Anterior view of abdominal muscles

Notice that in figure 7.1, the large rib cage and large pelvis are connected by the thin vertebral column. The abdominal muscles create a "basket weave" effect on the front of the body and wrap around the side of the body, so that when we stand erect or lift things or bend in all directions or walk, we are able to maintain our upright posture. The abdominals "hold us together" in a sense and give support to the vertebral column, trunk, and pelvis specifically.

There is a lot of attention paid in many yoga asana and fitness classes to the importance of the strength of the "core." But I feel that there is misunderstanding surrounding this topic in general.

I took a spinning class (stationary bicycling) not long ago, and the teacher, well-meaning no doubt, told us to "pull our abdominal muscles in to our backbone and keep them like that for the whole class to strengthen our core." I puckishly thought, "Okay, then I won't breathe."

The abdominal muscles, when strongly contracted, interfere with breathing. The abdominal muscles must be able to let go for us to breathe. I observed my abdominals frequently during class, and they seemed to know what to do all on their own. They helped to keep me up on the bike just fine, and they helped me exhale strongly when I needed to breathe quickly when things got very challenging.

Try this right now if you are able. Sit at the front of a stable chair with your feet securely on the floor. Put your hands so they firmly hold around your side waist. Now reach out with your right arm to the side so your arm is about parallel to the floor, and you are leaning to the right at about a 45° angle.

Do you feel your abdominal muscles contracting under your left hand? Of course this happens. It happens because it is necessary for the abdominal muscles to contract in order to stabilize, or hold, your trunk up and thus to prevent you from falling to the right and onto the floor. Did you have to tell them to contract? Of course not. Your abdominals "know" what to do to keep you upright against the force of gravity. They learned it as you began to sit up as a child. Your abdominal muscles are smarter than you are.

At the age of about six months, babies usually have developed enough trunk stability to sit up. At this age, they have something called "protective extension," but only to the front side of the body. This means that when the baby begins to fall forward in sitting, she naturally and quickly puts her arms straight in front of her to protect herself.

At eight months or so, protective extension now occurs to the side, and by about ten months, the baby has protective extension to the back. This gradual process of postural integration is normal, natural, and reflects, in no small measure, the abdominal muscles' ability to learn to respond so as to stabilize the baby's trunk and prevent possible injury. This learning is a pattern of action that includes other muscles as well. The nervous system of the baby is learning and remembering this whole pattern of muscular coordination among many muscles so that the net effect is trunk stabilization. The abdominals are the most important trunk stabilizer.

By the time we are adults, we pay little attention to the sophisticated postural interplay between the nervous system and the muscular system that keeps us upright. What I want for us to do as practitioners and teachers of yoga is to understand more about this interplay and, more importantly, how to facilitate it *naturally* without attempting to *control it from the intellectual mind*.

Our thinking mind is not able to control the intelligence of the abdominal muscles in yoga asana or in daily activities for that matter. If we had to tell ourselves how to walk across the room, we would never be able to make even the first step because of the very complex interplay that walking demands from our muscular and nervous systems, not to mention from our joints. We cannot use words to direct the specifics of movement because movement patterns, like the stabilization of the trunk, are much too unconscious and cannot be manipulated by our simple words and commands.

My hope is that what you learn in this chapter about your abdominal muscles and their importance in asana, and in all other types of movement, will make your life better and simpler. Join me as we learn how to "get out of the way" of the intrinsic intelligent action of our abdominals and be better able to challenge them in the most effective ways. *And that is not by doing sit-ups*; it is to challenge them in their function as stabilizers.

Your Structure

There are four abdominal muscles, and they work together like any team does, with integration and mutual support. The most superficial abdominal muscle is the rectus abdominis. "Rectus" means "a straight line," and this muscle runs in a straight line up the front of the trunk. It originates on the pubic bone and inserts on the cartilages of the fifth through seventh ribs, and on the end of the sternum at a structure called the xiphoid process.

You can easily feel the end of your breastbone at the top of your abdomen if you walk your fingers from the middle of your breastbone down where it ends at the abdomen. The rectus abdominis flexes the lumbar spine against gravity when the pelvis is fixed, and posteriorly tilts the pelvis when the rib cage is fixed. This muscle also assists with forced exhalation and increases intra-abdominal pressure when needed.

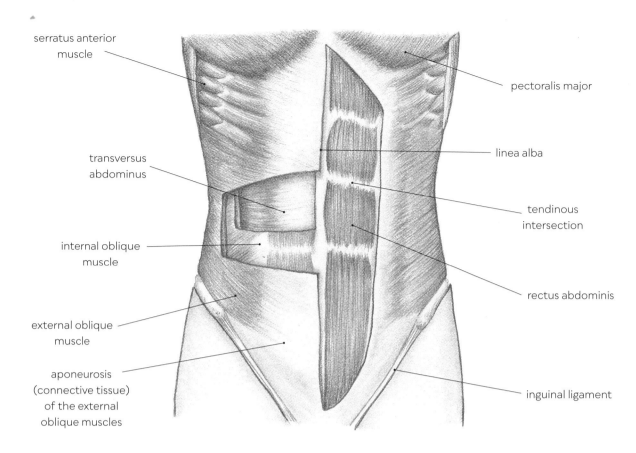

serratus anterior
muscle

pectoralis major

linea alba

transversus
abdominus

tendinous
intersection

internal oblique
muscle

external oblique
muscle

rectus abdominis

aponeurosis
(connective tissue)
of the external
oblique muscles

inguinal ligament

FIGURE 7.2

The next deeper layer of the abdominal muscles is made up of the external and internal oblique muscles. Observe their structure in figure 7.2. It is easy to see how these muscles mimic a "basket weave effect" around the sides of the abdomen.

The external obliques arise from the fifth to twelfth ribs and move downward and inward to attach to the outer iliac crest. The largest of the abdominal muscles, the external obliques, also attach to the xiphoid process, the connective tissue in the midline of the abdomen called the linea alba, the midclavicular line, and the pubic bones. Each external oblique helps you bend to the same side it is on and to rotate to the opposite side. Thus, the right external oblique helps you to side bend right and rotate left.

The internal obliques run perpendicular and deep to the external obliques and arise from the iliac crest, the inguinal ligament, and the thoracolumbar fascia. They move inward and upward and attach to the tenth through twelfth ribs and costal cartilages, the xiphoid process, the linea alba, and the pubic symphysis.

The internal obliques can help you forcefully exhale and side bend to the same side, but they rotate you to the same side as well. Thus, the right internal oblique helps you to side bend right *and* to rotate right. These muscles are sometimes called the "same-side rotators."

The final of the four abdominal muscles is the transverse abdominis. It is like a girdle around the front of the lower abdomen. It attaches to the costal cartilages of ribs seven through twelve, the lumbar fascia, the iliac crest, and the inguinal ligament. Its fibers run horizontally from the back to the front body and insert on the xiphoid process, linea alba, and pubic symphysis. It is an important stabilizer of the trunk, especially when lifting. Together with some of the erector muscles of the vertebral column, like the multifidus, the transverse abdominis can reduce as much as 40 percent of the pressure on the intervertebral discs in the back when it contracts during lifting.[5]

Even with just a short perusal of the anatomy of these four muscles, it becomes very obvious that strong abdominal muscles are important for our happy and healthy functioning as human beings. Let's learn how these muscles actually work together to help us practice asana.

Your Anatomy in Action

In the first section of this chapter, I left you with the statement that the best way to strengthen the abdominals is by using them as stabilizers. Before we continue to learn what this statement means in asana practice in the "Attentive Practice" section below, I would like for you to have an immediate experience of your abdominal muscles as stabilizers. You may want to just read this section and skip the actual positions if you are more than three months pregnant.

Please lie on your yoga mat on your back with your legs straight out on the floor. Rest for a breath or two. Now place one hand, palm down, over your navel. Inhale, and simply lift your head off the floor. Return your head to the floor. Now try it again. Both times I am sure that you felt something happening under your hand. Your abdominals were contracting.

Notice that you were not using them to flex your lumbar, like in tucking (flexing) the lumbar spine in standing. Instead, your abdominals were contracting to hold your rib cage and your pelvis together in a stable position. This is necessary for you to lift your head up against the force of gravity. Those who have had spinal cord damage at a level that paralyzes the nerves to the abdominal muscles cannot lift their heads off a pillow even though their neck muscles are normal and are still innervated by functioning nerves. For a muscle to act on a joint, it must cross that joint. But the abdominals do not cross from the trunk to the head, or neck, or attach there in any way.

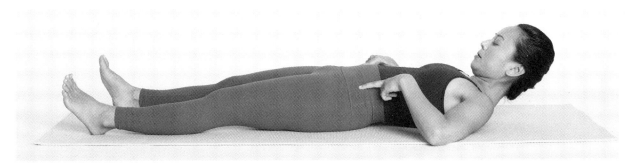

FIGURE 7.3

Abdominals are not neck flexors. They do, however, function in this example to prevent your rib cage from lifting up at the lower ribs so that your back arches and your pelvis tips. You will notice that your ribs and pelvis remain totally still while the neck moves into flexion when you try this simple movement.

Try this head-lifting exercise again. But this time place your thumbs on your lower ribs and your middle fingers on your ASIS.

Lift your head again and feel how your rib cage remains totally still. The abdominals are keeping it still so your normally weak neck flexors have better leverage to lift your head. This is the job of muscles that act in a stabilizing function; they make movement easier and more efficient by holding a body part still instead of moving a body part.

Now try one more time, but this time place a small firm pillow or a thin rolled blanket directly under your back bottom ribs so that they are lifted up and your back is arched.

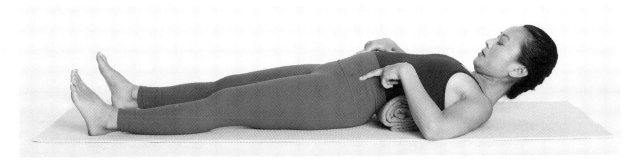

FIGURE 7.4

If this is uncomfortable for your lower back, skip this part of the experiment. Also skip this variation if you are more than twelve weeks pregnant. What is important to remember is that when your back is arched, your abdominals are stretched and are less able to provide the strength and stabilization they were able to before.

With this pillow under your back, your legs still straight, and your hands in the same position on ribs and ASIS, again try to lift your head. It will be possible but much harder. This is because by using the pillow and stretching your abdominals, you have made it hard for the abdominals to act as the stabilizers of the rib cage. This stabilization is necessary for the action of lifting your head to be efficient and relatively easy. The abdominals are important stabilizers for the trunk, and this stabilization affects the movement of the head, vertebral column, pelvis, arms, and legs as well.

There is another exercise we can explore to help you feel and understand your abdominals as stabilizers. Please get down on your yoga mat on all fours. Make sure your thighs and arms are in an exact vertical position and take care of your wrists by making sure that before you go any further, your palms are directly under your shoulder joints, and your whole arm is exactly in a vertical line.

Lift your right arm up parallel to the floor so your right hand is higher than your shoulder. Keep your arm straight. Now simply move your weight slightly forward. You will immediately feel your abdominals contract to stabilize your trunk and hold you up against the ever-present force of gravity, which is acting to pull your body down.

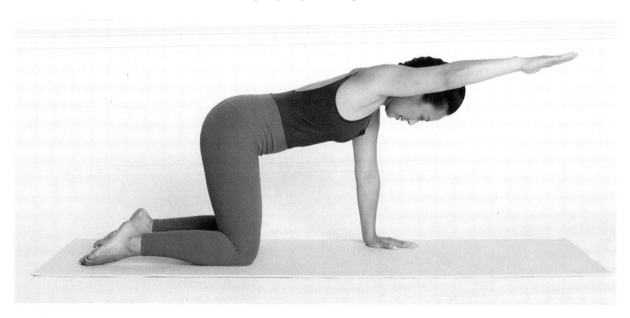

FIGURE 7.5

Stay a while. Keep breathing. Try moving a little farther forward. The longer you stay, the more you will be aware of your abdominal muscles contracting. This will definitely be getting harder and harder. Come down as needed. Try it with the other arm.

There will be a little shift of your trunk to the left when you lift your right arm, as well as the opposite when you lift your left arm. This is natural and fine, but be careful not to twist or rotate your trunk. Keep your trunk level as much as you can and make sure as well that your hand does not drift down below the level of your shoulder. And by all means, breathe.

I like to teach this, and similar positions, both to help students challenge their abdominals and strengthen them as stabilizers and to show them that sit-ups are really not as effective. Many people can do a lot of sit-ups, but most students find that the type of position described above gets challenging must faster than sit-ups.

My understanding is that if we want to strengthen any muscle, we must do so by making that muscle work against gravity during a movement that challenges its main function. Muscles sometimes have multiple actions, but there is always a main one. Here's an interesting example of that principle.

Let's look at the biceps brachii, the large muscle in the front compartment of the upper arm,

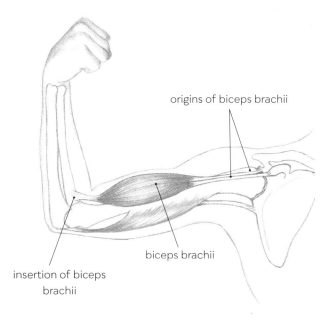

origins of biceps brachii

biceps brachii

insertion of biceps brachii

FIGURE 7.6

and what I sometimes call the "body-builder muscle" because it is so often shown in ads and pictures for gyms and fitness facilities.

Most people think that the main action of the biceps is to flex or bend the elbow. Actually, the main action of the biceps brachii is to supinate the forearm. Supination is the act of turning the palm up. With your arm at your side, keep your upper arm still and bend your elbow to a 90° angle with your palm facing downward. Now turn your palm up; that movement is called supination. I help my students remember the name of this action of the elbow by telling them to think of carrying a bowl of soup, which is done with palms upward.

Here's our experiment. Flex your right elbow with your palm down, in other words, in pronation. Now reach across your body with your left hand and hold firmly on to the biggest part of your right biceps. Imagine that Ganesha, the elephant deity in the Hindu pantheon, is sitting on the back of your palm. This is an image to help you create resistance to the flexion of your elbow.

Try to lift Ganesha by flexing your elbow joint. At the same time, create resistance to this movement so you make the muscle work hard. Feel and gauge how much your biceps fibers contract in flexion in pronation.

Let go, and now, keeping your elbow in flexion, turn your forearm so that your palm faces upward; this is called supination. Again, invite the imaginary Ganesha to help, this time by sitting in the palm your hand. Remember, he is very heavy. Try to do the difficult job of flexing your elbow joint and lifting your forearm and Ganesha. Flex against the tremendous imaginary weight of Ganesha in supination. Keep everything else still.

Don't forget to hold on to the biggest part of your biceps with your left hand during this contraction. I think you will be surprised to feel how much more your biceps works to flex the elbow with the forearm in supination than it does trying to flex the elbow in pronation. The biceps is better able to recruit more muscle fibers when you flex the elbow in supination.

This is because the primary action of the biceps brachii is supination, followed by elbow flexion, and finally shoulder flexion. This is why it is so much easier to do a chin-up in supination than it is to do a pull-up in pronation. The biceps brachii is much more effective in elbow flexion when you ask it to supinate at the same time.

There is a similar truth about the abdominals. You definitely use the abdominals in sit-ups, but the abdominals first function is stabilization. Thus, it makes sense to me to challenge the abdominals with stabilization instead of sit-ups. Certainly, trying to tuck the tailbone in Mountain Pose while telling your abdominal muscles to contract is not an efficient strengthening technique either. In Mountain Pose, the abdominals, while important for helping with the upright posture, are not what primarily holds you up. It is mostly a balancing pose of the pelvis on the head of the femurs, with added stability offered by the hip muscles, knee joints and muscles, and other leg muscles.

MAIN POINTS TO REMEMBER FROM THIS CHAPTER

→ The main function of the abdominal muscles in movement is the stabilization of the trunk.

→ Muscles are more effective when performing their main action.

→ Trust your abdominals to function intelligently when you challenge them as stabilizers against gravity.

Attentive Practice

In this section we will practice asana that are useful in strengthening your abdominal muscles, but paradoxically, I would like to add a word here about stretching the abdominal muscles. I suggest that when you do any kind of a backbend, you intentionally let go of your abdominal muscles and let them stretch. If you try to tighten the abdominal muscles in a backbend, two things will happen.

First, it will be difficult because you are first asking them to let go and then telling them not to; you are telling them to contract. If you are stretching your abdominals, then simple stretch them. Do not confuse contracting the abdominals in a pose like Cobra Pose with strengthening the abdominals.

Second, contracting the abdominals in a backbend is not very helpful for protecting the back. When you contract your abdominals in Cobra Pose, what you are really doing is just coming out of the pose some. Better to simply do less of a bend and keep the abdominals soft and free to be stretched.

CAUTIONS

With the exception of Tree Pose (Vrksasana), I do not recommend that you practice the poses presented in this section after the third month of pregnancy. As the baby grows, the abdominals become more and more stretched, as do other soft tissues of the abdomen. The pregnant abdomen may feel "toned" to the touch, but even though it feels strong, it could be weaker than you think. Take care.

In order to strengthen a muscle, we must ask it to do a little bit more than it is used to doing. So, proceed slowly and pay attention to your own limits. If you feel sore the day after you practice poses to strengthen your abdominal muscles, rest a day or two and then begin again, challenging yourself a little bit less this time, and build gradually to a stronger practice.

PROPS NEEDED

- Nonslip yoga mat
- Yoga blanket

Tree Pose

VRKSASANA

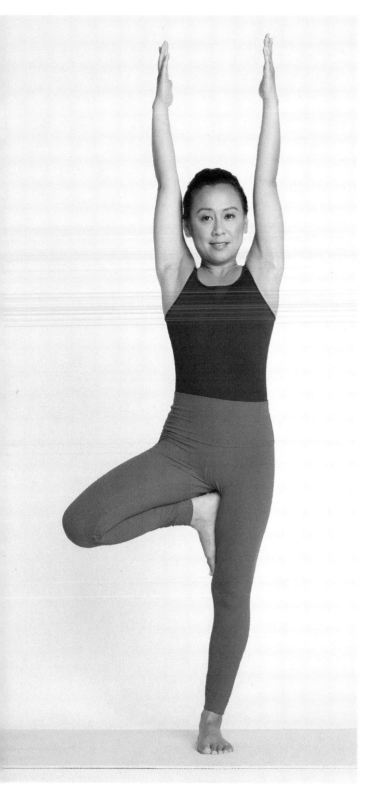

Stand on your yoga mat. It is better to have bare feet. Start in Mountain Pose (see chapter 1, page 11). Put your hands around your waist. Now lift your right foot off the ground and place it in front of you as if to take a step.

Notice that the moment you lift your knee, you not only shift your weight onto your left leg, you also contract your abdominal muscles. They are now acting as stabilizers to hold your trunk stable and safe. This is what they do with every step we take. The abdominals keep us upright when we are vertical and moving.

Now, with an exhalation, bring your right foot toward the left inner groin, and with the help of your hands, place it there, toes pointing down.

When your foot is securely in place and pressing into your inner leg, inhale as you take your arms out to the side and stretch them over your head. Keep the arms straight and let your shoulder blades move up naturally. Fix your eyes on a point on the floor a few feet in front of you. Keep the breath soft and moving. After a few breaths, come out of the pose. Practice it on the other side.

When this pose has become familiar, try it a foot from the wall, with your back facing the wall. Then partially or fully close your eyes and observe how much visual cues help your balance. When they close their eyes, most people find that they are much more wobbly. Notice that your ankle and foot are a bigger part of your awareness in the pose as they accommodate somewhat quickly to minute changes in your balance. Now open your eyes and observe if your balance becomes easier. Be sure to do both sides.

FIGURE 7.7

Plank Pose

CHATURANGA DANDASANA 1

Get down on your hands and knees on your mat. Now straighten your arms and legs. Make sure that the center of your wrist is directly underneath your shoulder joint and that you are standing on the balls of your feet with your feet about ten inches apart.

Slightly drop your chin so the head comes into line with the rest of the body. Lift your thoracic spine (mid-back) up above the level of the shoulder blades. Tuck your tailbone under and lift with your navel. Breathe. (See figure 5.17 on page 89.)

You might find it surprising that I am instructing you now to tuck in the pose, because I was so adamant about *not* tucking in chapter 1, However, there I was instructing you on how to do Mountain Pose. There is a completely different relationship between the body and gravity in Mountain Pose and the body and gravity in Plank Pose.

In Plank Pose, gravity is pulling directly down on the entire surface of the back body. We are asking our body to hold itself up against this force. We now need the abdominals to work to help keep us from collapsing. When the abdominals contract, they flex the vertebral column, or attempt to flex it.

If you allow yourself to arch your lumbar in this pose, to drop your breastbone and hang the thoracic spine down between the shoulder blades as shown in figure 7.8, you will find it harder. This is because when your entire vertebral column is arched, it is harder for the abdominals to contract and stabilize you.

Remember to lift up in the pose: from the breastbone, from the mid-back, from the abdomen. This not only will make the pose easier and more effective for abdominal strengthening, but you will also no doubt enjoy it more because you are working with your body's natural intelligence instead of against it.

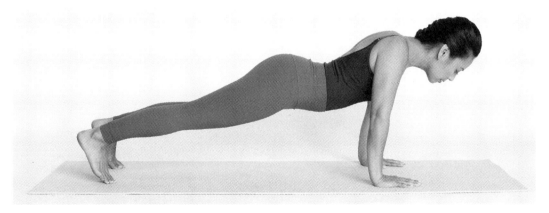

FIGURE 7.8

Side Plank Pose

VASISTHASANA

To practice this pose, get on your mat and take Plank Pose. In this variation, separate your feet a little farther apart than in the previous pose.

Keeping the breath soft and moving, begin to lift your right arm up and turn your body so that you are balancing on your left arm only.

Make sure that your left arm is exactly vertical and that your wrist is directly under your left shoulder socket. Experiment a bit to see which hand position feels best. Some students like their fingers pointing straight ahead as is shown in the photo.

Notice that the model in figure 7.9 is turned onto the sides of her feet and not onto the soles. To do this, make sure that there is enough room for your

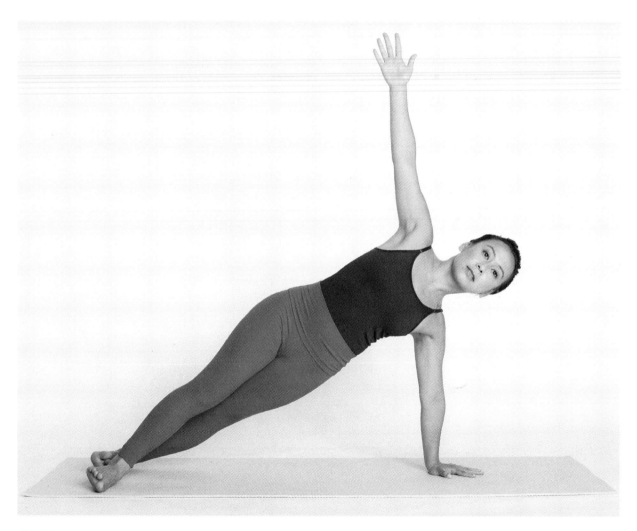

FIGURE 7.9

feet. Usually this pose is taught with the feet held together, but I find the foot position shown here makes balancing easier so that the focus can be on the abdomen.

Once you are in the pose, lift up from your waist. Imagine that your waist is higher than your pelvis. Do not let yourself sag down. This position of lifting will engage the abdominals. Come down, rest, and then try it again. Then practice this pose with the right arm supporting you. You can also vary the pose by doing it on your forearms. You may find this variation more difficult.

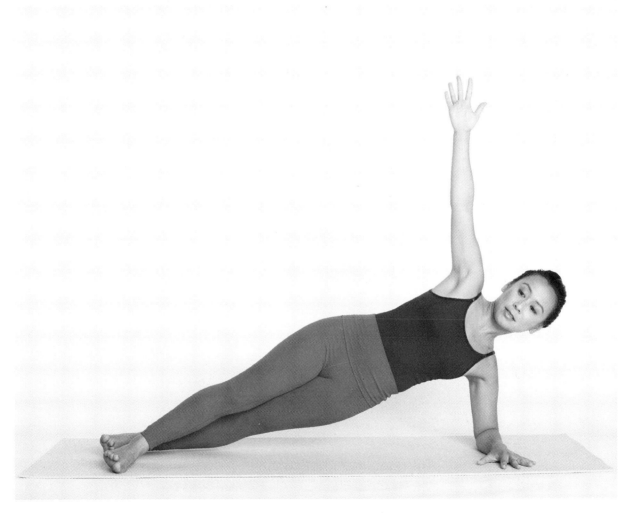

FIGURE 7.10

Boat Pose

NAVASANA

At the beginning of this chapter, I told a story about my first attempt at Boat Pose. Here is the way I discovered to practice it so that I liked it, and it helped me protect my back and strengthen my abdominals at the same time.

Sit on your mat on a folded blanket. This is especially useful if you have a prominent coccyx bone, as many students do.

Begin by bending your knees, and as you lean backward, hold the back of each knee with a hand.

Notice that if you rock forward, you are sitting in front of your sitting bones, and that will make you arch your lower back. If you rock backward some, you will notice that you are now sitting on your lower sacrum instead. The more comfortable place to sit is on the lower sacrum.

Once you have rocked back, begin to find your balance. Be sure to keep your knees bent at first. Once you have found your balance, slowly straighten your right leg so that your right tibia is parallel to the floor. Do the same with your left. Now release your hands and balance. Straighten your arms in front of you, with your palms turned inward. This is step one.

Make sure you keep your lower abdomen concave. That means your lower back is rounded. This position will give your abdominal muscles the ability to contract to help you stay up. If you sit in front of your sitting bones and are arched, your abdominals will be stretched and not at a mechanical advantage for stabilizing your trunk.

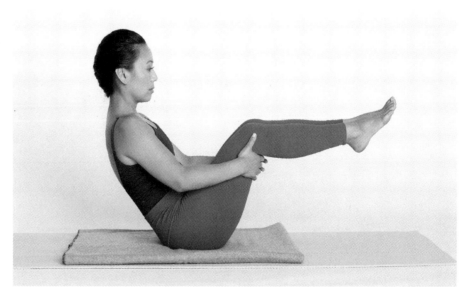

FIGURE 7.11

If you are arched in Boat Pose, your thighs will begin to talk to you. Because you have limited the ability of the abdominals to hold you up, the quadriceps, and other muscles with the ability to help with hip flexion, will be working quite hard.

Instead, if you let your lower back round, or think of pulling your lower ribs inward and drawing the side tops of your pelvis toward each other, it will help. Then the abdominals, which only can work well in flexion of the hips and vertebral column, will be able to do what they are designed to do: stabilize your trunk.

Notice that even if there is a slight rounding in the vertebral column, the model's upper back is not "collapsing." In fact, it is softly open. There is much more ease in this way of practicing the pose.

The final stage is to straighten both legs.

This can be difficult for people with long legs because the leverage is wrong. Offer yourself and your students the option of Boat Pose with the shins parallel to the floor. This is much safer for the lower back for taller people and is still a great strengthener of the abdominal muscles.

Whichever way you position the legs in the pose, remember to breath and enjoy yourself. Kids especially seem to like trying this pose. But since kids tend to have weak abdominals, teach it to them with bent knees only.

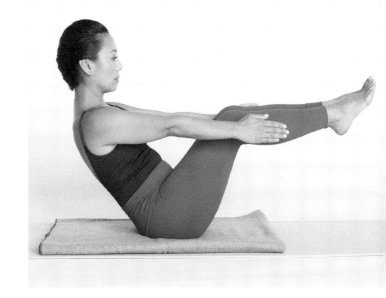

FIGURE 7.12

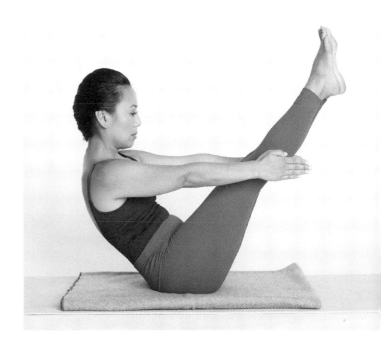

FIGURE 7.13

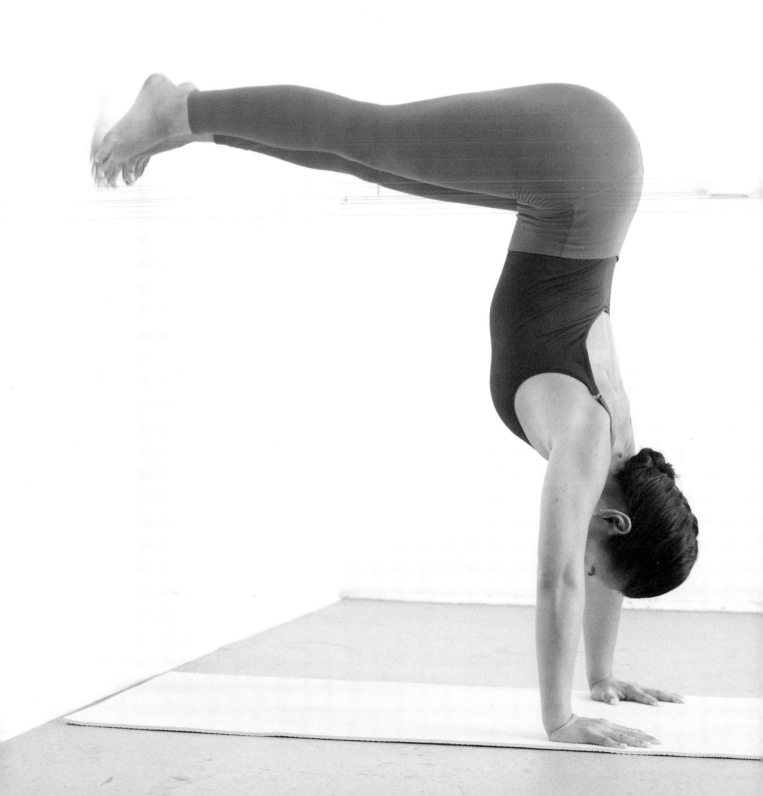

8

Upside Down

HEAD, NECK, HANDS, AND ELBOWS

When I am upside down, I gain a new perspective on the world and my place in it.

ONE OF THE UNIQUE POSITIONS in the practice of yoga asana is that of being upside down. I actually learned my first inversion, a headstand, from my mother. She had been athletic during her youth, winning a tennis scholarship to university at the age of sixteen.

When I was growing up, we would sometimes all sit out in the yard in the delightful summer evening coolness and watch the stars appear. I remember that more than once she challenged me to stand on my head with her. She would carefully place her head on the grass, position her hands to create a tripod shape, and then walk her feet in, bending her knees to her chest. Then she would tip backward to find her balance as her feet left the ground, and finally go up, straightening her legs to balance there for a few seconds in a perfect vertical line.

My friends from the block and I were very impressed, and I eventually learned to do a headstand with an air of nonchalance, as if all kids did headstands with their mother in the front yard.

So years later when I started the practice of asana, Headstand (Sirsasana) did not seem strange or scary to me. I found that there were differences between a headstand in yoga class and the way I learned it from my mother. The first difference was the way we placed our hands, and because of this different position, I found that I could stay up longer in the pose in yoga class. The other difference was that we were taught lots of variations in leg and trunk positions to practice while holding the pose.

There were other inversions in yoga asana class as well, and I eventually learned about the benefits of these inversions and how to practice them with care and patience. In most cases, so can you. But in order to do so, it is necessary to undertake the practice of inversions with respect and knowledge. Too often I have seen or heard of yoga students practicing Headstand with little or no preparation. I have seen students practice Shoulder Stand with no blankets, putting too much weight on the lower cervical and upper thoracic vertebrae while strongly reversing their normal curves. In fact, I have actually seen students who have developed callouses on the skin that covers the bony prominences of the vertebrae of the neck from this way of practicing.

I want to share with you in this chapter how you might learn inversions in a way that avoids such yoga myths as "there is only one position for the head to take in Headstand" or "the palms of the hands need to be completely flat on the floor in Handstand." We will address these issues later in this chapter.

My favorite yoga myth is "inversions bring more blood to the brain." Not so. In fact, the amount of blood in the brain is strongly regulated to remain at a very constant level. Anyone who has stood still long enough to get dizzy and then pass out can affirm this physiological truth.

If the blood pressure in the brain drops it can cause you to pass out, which is the body's solution to putting you in a horizontal position so that more blood can reach your brain. It is actually the oxygen the blood carries that the brain craves because of its high metabolic rate. Therefore, the brain requires a steady and even quantity of blood/oxygen to function well whether you are sound asleep or running a marathon.

So let's begin to study inversions in general, and some in particular. Hopefully this study will help you determine if and when to practice inversions, as well as instruct you in how to do them safely and enjoyably.

Why You Need to Know This

Mostly when we think about a yoga pose, we think about its physical shape. Is it a forward bend? A backbend? A twist? But traditional wisdom teaches that a yoga asana is not only a physical shape that the body can express, but it also has deep effects on the mind, the psyche, and the state of the subtle energy in our body.

Traditional wisdom also teaches that inversions can have a powerful effect on our balance, both physical and mental, as well as the perspective of how we view the world. I remember as a child lying on my back and hanging off the edge of my parents' bed. My brother and I would lie there and look at the ceiling, imagining that it was the floor. We would laugh when we saw a family member walk by, because it seemed that the "floor" they were walking on looked like the ceiling to us. How funny to see our dad walking on the "ceiling."

I personally believe that inversions lie at the very heart of yoga asana practice and, furthermore, that there is almost always a modification for an inversion that can be created so as to make some variation of an inverted pose possible for almost all students.

Inversions, in some form, need to be part of most students' practice. Inversions affect the blood flow in the body, although the amount of blood in the brain stays steady remember, whether we are standing on our feet, our hands, our shoulders, or our head. Inversions can directly benefit the heart by increasing the amount of blood the heart receives, which is called cardiac return, during the holding of an inversion. This usually causes the heart to slow down and therefore rest.

Some of my women students also report that regular practice of especially Shoulder Stand Pose and Plough Pose (Halasana) have helped them to reduce the frequency and severity of the hot flashes sometimes associated with perimenopause. At the very least, the stillness and internalization of focus one has in inversions can help to reduce stress, anxiety, swelling in the legs, and blood pressure.

So what is an inversion exactly? My definition is that an inversion is a pose in which the head is lower than the heart. This would include such poses as Standing Forward Bend, Wide-Legged Forward Bend (Prasarita Padottanasana), Downward-Facing Dog Pose, Bridge Pose (Setu Bandhasana), both supported and active, as well as Headstand, Legs-Up-the-Wall Pose (Viparita Karani), Supported Shoulder Stand, Plough Pose, Elbow Stand (Pincha Mayurasana), and Handstand (Adho Mukha Vrksasana).

I think of inversions as being classified in two broad categories. The first category is an inversion where the head, but not necessarily all of the rest of the body, is below the heart. These would be inversions that are created in some of the standing poses. Downward-Facing Dog Pose and Bridge Pose also belong to this first category and are generally more accessible for a wider number of students. These poses can help you prepare for the second category of poses, if, and only if, they are appropriate for you.

The second category is made up of more advanced inversions that we hold for longer periods of time, like Headstand, Half Shoulder Stand, Shoulder Stand, Plough Pose, Elbow Stand, and Handstand. These poses require more strength and flexibility and should be practiced only under the supervision of a well-seasoned teacher who can give each student some individual attention during the learning process.

The two poses from this second group that are most central to the practice of inversions are Headstand and Shoulder Stand. I consider these two poses, sometimes referred to respectively as the King and Queen of poses, to be at the very center of yoga asana practice, in part because they are traditionally held for longer periods of time than other inversions, and they seem to have the most powerful effects of all the inversions in yoga asana practice.

Later in the chapter, there will be instructions for practicing two poses from the first category of inversions—Standing Forward Bend and Wide-Legged Forward Bend—but in this chapter, I want to focus specifically on two poses from the second category: Headstand and Handstand. In so doing, we will put our attention on the head and neck for Headstand and on the hands and wrists for Handstand. For this reason, please review page 32 in chapter 2 for instructions on practicing Supported Shoulder Stand, as it will not be covered again in this chapter.

Your Structure

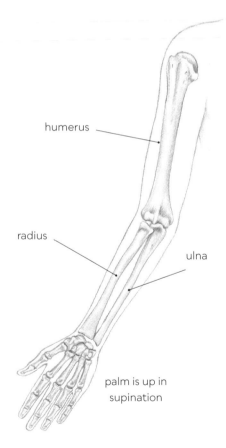

FIGURE 8.1
Anterior view of right upper extremity

humerus

radius

ulna

palm is up in supination

Inversions usually involve some weight-bearing on the head, neck, shoulders, forearms, or hands. Please review the anatomy of the neck in chapter 2 (see page 21) and the anatomy of the shoulder joint in chapter 5 (see page 76). This review will make the instructions in the "Attentive Practice" section of this chapter easier to understand. Because we have already discussed the shoulder joint, here we will begin with the anatomy of the forearm, wrist, and hand to round out our study of the upper extremity.

One of the most obvious things to know about the forearms, hands, and wrists is that they are not normally weight-bearing. This is not to say that they *cannot* bear weight, but rather that weight-bearing is not their primary function. The lower extremities are made for the primary functions of weight-bearing and locomotion. So if we are to bear weight on the upper extremity, let us do so with knowledge and awareness.

The radius, the ulna, and the humerus make up the elbow joint.

Notice the long slender bones of the forearm, the radius, and the ulna.

Note that the ulna curves under to join with the humerus on the posterior side of the elbow joint. Of the two forearm bones, it is the lesser mobile.

However, the radius attaches to the humerus in a different way from the ulna, and this makes it more mobile. The radius has the ability to cross over the ulna during the movement called pronation. Remember that even when the radius moves over the ulna when you turn your palm down, or pronate your forearm, the radius is always on the thumb side of your forearm. No matter what position your forearm is in, the radius always remains on the thumb side. Try moving your forearm around, palm up or palm down, and you can always use your other hand to feel the radius is on the thumb side.

To feel the radiating, or crossing-over, action of the radius, do this. Sit upright with your right elbow joint at 90° of flexion. This means that your elbow joint is about halfway bent toward your shoulder and that the bones of the forearm are parallel to the floor. Turn your palm up.

Now with the fingers of your left hand, reach across your body and hold your forearm quite firmly at a point about six inches up from your wrist and try to feel the bones. If you are having difficulty feeling your radius (on the outside, or lateral side), find a slightly different location on your forearm to try this experiment.

Once you have found a location on your forearm without too much flesh where you can easily feel both the radius and the ulna, squeeze your fingers and pronate your forearm, i.e., turn your palm down. If you pay attention, you will definitely feel your radius moving over your ulna so the bones are now crossed. Try this a couple of times. We will discuss this ability to rotate and what it means for weight-bearing more in the next section.

At the distal end of the radius and the ulna are the eight carpal bones. These small bones articulate with the radius and ulna and with the metacarpals, or bones of the hand. Finally, the metacarpals join with the phalanges, the bones of the fingers.

The radius has a very different relationship with the carpal bones than does the ulna. At the articulation of the radius and the carpals, you can see how the radius continues farther than the ulna. Because of this, when people fall down on a hard surface and catch themselves with their hand, the radius absorbs most of the impact of the fall. Thus, we are more likely to fracture the distal radius than the distal ulna with falls.

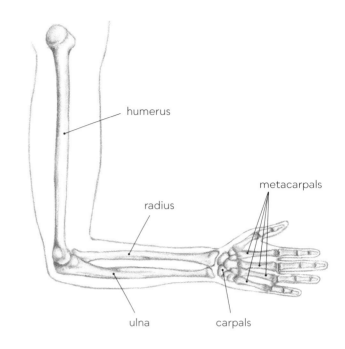

FIGURE 8.2

The extension of the wrist, which is bringing the back of the hand toward the forearm, has a greater range than flexion, which is bringing the palm toward the forearm. The muscles that flex the wrist are located on the surface of the forearm that you can see when you are in supination. The muscles that extend the wrist are located on the surface of the forearm that you can see when you are in pronation.

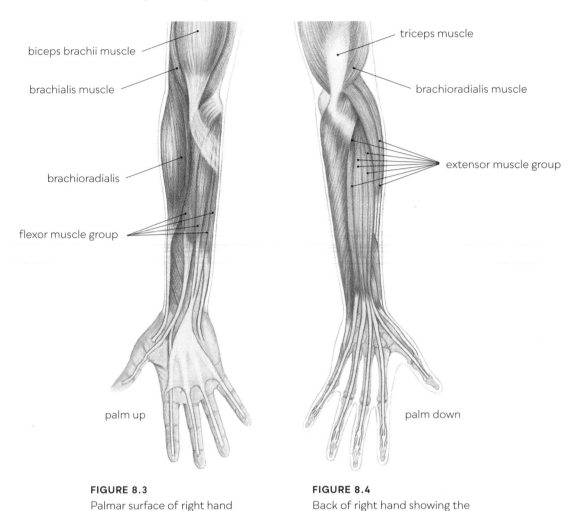

biceps brachii muscle

brachialis muscle

brachioradialis

flexor muscle group

triceps muscle

brachioradialis muscle

extensor muscle group

palm up

palm down

FIGURE 8.3
Palmar surface of right hand showing wrist flexor muscles

FIGURE 8.4
Back of right hand showing the wrist extensor muscles

You can feel this distinction easily. While sitting at a sturdy table, pronate your right forearm and bend your elbow to 90° of flexion. Now place your hand under the table so the back of your hand is comfortably pressing against the underside of the table. Place your left palm on the upper third of your right forearm. Now try to extend your right wrist, i.e., try to bring your wrist up toward the ceiling into extension. Push firmly with your hand against the table. Notice how the muscles on the pronator side of your forearm are contracting, trying to extend the wrist against the challenge of the table.

Now try this same experiment with your forearm supinated. This time try to lift the wrist up into flexion against the table. You will now feel the wrist flexor muscles on the supination side of the forearm contracting strongly.

It turns out that movement patterns in the upper extremity tend to link pronation of the forearm with extension of the elbow joint, and supination of the forearm with flexion of the elbow. This understanding will come in handy when following the instructions given below for Downward-Facing Dog Pose, Headstand, Handstand, and Elbow Stand.

Notice how much smaller all the bones and joints of the upper extremity are than the bones and joints of your lower leg, ankle, and foot. Turn your hand over and look at your palm.

Do you see the arch there? It is not as large or as strong as the arches in your feet. The feet have several arches to facilitate the distribution of weight to help to provide balance in standing, as well as to help create the proper propulsion needed in walking, and especially in running.

The hand is not nearly as powerful as the foot, and certainly not nearly as well prepared to bear weight. With a little observation, it is easy to understand the need for attention when we ask the hands and wrists to bear our whole body's weight.

Your Anatomy in Action

We have already discussed Downward-Facing Dog Pose twice. The first mention was in chapter 5 when we discussed the shoulders in the pose (see page 86); the second mention was in chapter 6 in relationship to the knees in the pose (see page 107). Here we will discuss the position of the whole arm, wrist, hand, and fingers.

When practicing Downward-Facing Dog Pose, the hands are assuredly bearing weight, but that weight is not directly straight down onto the wrists and hands in a vertical line. This makes weight-bearing a little less dramatic for these structures than in Handstand. However, it is nonetheless important to know how to distribute the weight in a way that protects the wrists.

Stand beside a heavy table and place your hands, palms down, on that table, slightly wider than shoulder width apart, with your middle fingers pointing exactly straight ahead. Now lean forward against the table and place strong weight on your hands. If you have any pain in your wrists, skip this experiment.

Notice that you likely tend to roll outward on your hands, so that the weight is more toward your little finger than your thumb. When you do this, you also may notice that your elbows tend to bend.

Now roll the weight to the thumb side of your hand, where there is more stability in the wrist. Feel the weight at the base of your thumb and at the first joint of the index finger that is nearest the palm. Make sure your thumb is stretched out to the side and firmly pressing the surface. Your elbows will straighten, the muscles along your entire arm will become active, and likely your wrist will feel much better.

Keeping your hands in this position, begin to walk backward from the table so that your trunk is slowly moving down toward the floor. But keep your focus on the thumb side of your hand and root of your index finger pressing down. Notice as you walk slowly backward that your entire arm is internally rotating, exactly as was discussed in chapter 5 on the shoulder joint action in Downward-Facing Dog Pose. The next time you practice Downward-Facing Dog Pose, use this exact hand position to create both freedom and stability in your hand and wrist.

The hand and wrist position will be slightly different for Handstand. What has changed? What has changed is your position relative to gravity. In Handstand, the weight of the pose is directly down onto your hands and not diagonally dispersed like in Downward-Facing Dog Pose.

So, the hand position needs to be different to accommodate the extra weight that the hand and wrist are being asked to bear. To feel this, get down on your hands and knees on your yoga mat. Now lean forward over your wrists and notice how it feels if you try to flatten your palms to the floor like is often taught in yoga asana class.

Instead, first remember that the feet, whose main job is weight-bearing, have several arches. Since weight-bearing is not the main function of the hand, wouldn't it make sense to create an arch in your hand during weight-bearing so that your hand more resembles the foot? Remember, in the body, form is created by function, and function shapes the form.

To create an arch, with your hands flat on the floor, pull the pads of your fingers toward you so now the fingers are arched, your palm is arched, and it is only the rim of your hand that is on the floor. For some people it helps if they imagine holding a basketball in their palms. Now lean forward and place weight on your hands. Voilà! The weight is now spread more evenly around the rim of your hand, and the wrist is much happier. In addition, when you actually practice Handstand, you will better be able to balance.

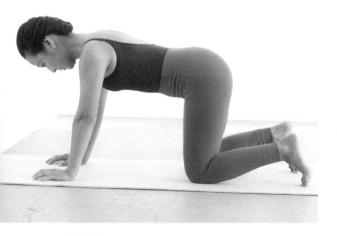

FIGURE 8.5

This is because with an arch, you can make the same kind of micromovements to balance as you do when standing on your feet. You probably don't realize you are making these micromovements to stay upright, but you are. These micromovements are called postural sway. This is the process of your body making continual and slight adjustments to gravity, moment to moment.

Creating a hand position that resembles the arches in the feet makes balancing dynamic, more adaptable, and easier. And it is better for the wrist and hand than trying to flatten the palm because of a yoga myth that does not reflect the actual anatomy of the area.

No teacher tells their students to try to flatten the arches of the feet in standing poses; quite the contrary, teachers want their students to have normal arches in the feet because normal arches allow for better biomechanical movements in the feet, ankles, knees, hips, and spine. Follow the wisdom of your body and create an arch in your hand when weight-bearing in Handstand and in other arm balances where the weight is on the hands.

A more advanced inversion is Elbow Stand, and it requires not only strength, but also attention to the placement of the elbows, forearms, wrists, and hands on the mat.

The most important aspect of your relationship with your mat in this pose is stability. It is easier to balance away from the wall in this pose because there is a greater area of support created by the fact that the body weight is spread over the forearms and hands. This is a greater weight-bearing surface than that on the forearms in Handstand when you just stand on your hands and the edge of the forearms.

A common placement of the hands and elbows is one in which the elbows are allowed to move outward, wider than the shoulders. When this happens, the hands come inward so you are now creating a triangular shape with your arms.

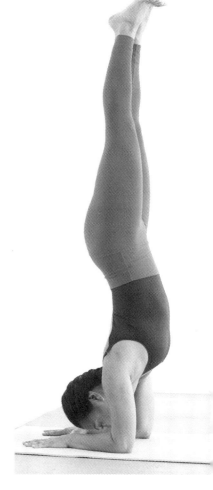

FIGURE 8.6

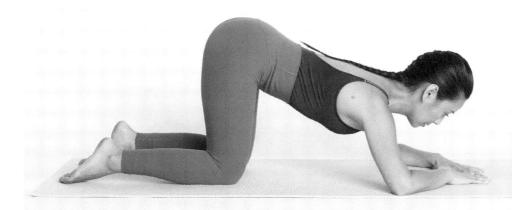

FIGURE 8.7

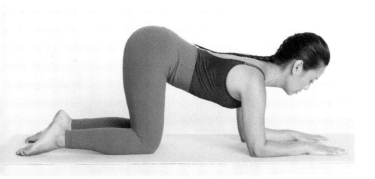

FIGURE 8.8

This position is counterproductive because the humerus is no longer vertical; when the humerus is vertical, there is more congruence at the shoulder joint. As mentioned previously in this book, the greater the congruence between two joint surfaces, the greater the stability in the joint. When Elbow Stand is practiced with a vertical humerus, the glenoid fossa and the head of the humerus have more congruence and thus more stability. Not only will this make practicing the pose more stable, it will also make balancing easier.

To feel this difference, get onto your yoga mat on all fours. Now come down onto your forearms and place them in a triangular position with your elbows out farther than your shoulders, and the tips of your thumbs and index fingers touching. Now lean forward or straighten your legs a bit and place weight on your whole upper extremity.

Try again and this time, first place your elbows directly under your shoulder joints; keep your elbows bent while you do this. Now turn your palms toward your face and lay your right forearm on the floor. Roll slowly into pronation and at the same time push outward slightly on the ulna bone so that all the forearm flesh is forced toward the inside of your forearm.

Once you have finished pronation, notice that you feel very much in contact with the mat with both forearm bones. If you just set your forearm down on the floor, your contact with the mat will feel "wiggly" and not firmly in contact with the mat.

Now do the same positioning with your left forearm and then straighten your legs so you can put weight on your forearms. Take care not to allow your elbows to move outward; keep them still. Push down some more on the elbow and the base of the root of the thumb and straighten your legs.

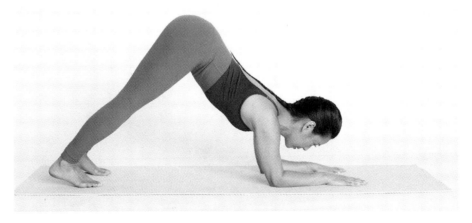

FIGURE 8.9

Remember that you have more power to extend the elbow when you are pronating. And keeping your elbows directly under your shoulder joints allows the pectoralis muscles in the upper chest to adduct (move toward the midline) your humerus bones (see figure 8.9 above). These strong muscles will give stability to the front of your chest in the pose. Keeping a pristine alignment of the upper and lower arms and the hands will require focus, but in the end will be worth it. Keeping your humerus bones exactly vertical will allow the force of gravity to move down your upper arms and that, accompanied by the pushing down action facilitated by pronation, will create the base of the pose. Be sure to review these instructions before you practice the full pose that is taught in the "Attentive Practice" section below.

The position for the upper extremity in Headstand is somewhat more complicated than its position in Elbow Stand because Headstand demands more from the finger and wrist positions. Additionally, the relationship between the head and the hands is most critical to practicing a safe and happy Headstand.

Try the beginning of Headstand as instructed below only if it is a wise decision for your neck and wise for you to practice an inversion. Please read the contraindications to Headstand offered in the beginning of the "Attentive Practice" section below. Always err on the side of caution.

Once again step onto your mat and start by positioning yourself on all fours. Just as with Forearm Stand, carefully place your elbows exactly underneath your shoulder joints so the upper bones of your arms are exactly vertical.

As with Elbow Stand, place your forearms on the mat in supination.

Begin to press your forearms firmly into the mat and turn your hands so that your palms face each other. Now push your ulna outward so you feel the full length of the ulnar bone firmly on the mat. When you do this, notice that this movement makes all the flesh on the forearm move toward the inside

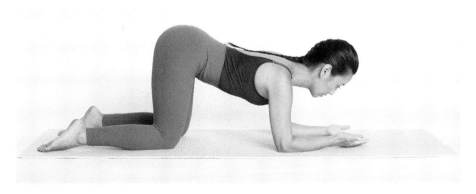

FIGURE 8.10

of your arms. Now lift your hands, and one at a time move the little finger side of each hand to the floor so that you feel the bones of the hand pressing firmly on the floor. Finally turn your palms to face each other. Now interlock your fingers all the way so that the root of your fingers, called the web spaces, are firmly touching.

Lean forward and put some weight on your forearms. This weight should feel stable and comfortable. Slightly release the little fingers and ring fingers apart now, about half an inch or so, so that your palms and wrists are exactly vertical.

Here's why I suggest this action. Sit back and look at your right palm. Notice the angle that is created by drawing an imaginary line from the base of your index finger to the outer edge of the little finger.

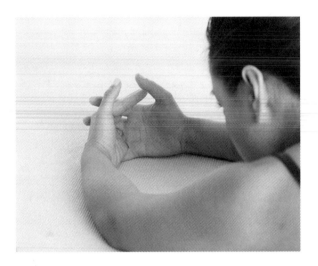

FIGURE 8.11

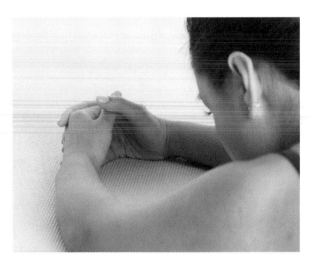

FIGURE 8.12

The line is straight from the index to the ring finger but suddenly drops in a downward angle at the little finger. If you push all the fingers together evenly when they are intertwined, you will find that you are turning your wrist outward, i.e., supinating your forearms. Move the little finger and ring finger web spaces, those spaces between the roots of the fingers, a little apart so that there is a vertical line along the root of your fingers

Remember that in supination, it is harder to extend your elbow with as much power as when you are in pronation. When you are in Headstand, you are pushing the earth away from you. In effect, you are trying to extend your elbow, even though the joint doesn't move. You are contracting the muscles you need to push downward strongly. Contracting a muscle in a manner that does not change its length is called an isometric contraction.

The word *isometric* comes from the Greek *isos* meaning "equal" and *metron* meaning "a measure" or "having equal measurement." So, there is no change in the angle of the elbow, but the triceps muscles are nonetheless contracting to try to straighten it. You can feel a similar isometric type contraction in standing if you bend your knees almost halfway and hold the position. Your quadriceps muscles in the front of your thighs are undergoing an isometric contraction to hold you upright.

This function of muscles is called stabilization. The pronator muscles of the forearm and other shoulder and upper extremity muscles are stabilizing your shoulder joint to allow you to use the upper extremity and head to stand on, thus Headstand.

Resume the hand position described above with your fingers interlocked, your wrists slightly turning inward, and the weight firmly and pleasantly full on your ulna bones. Lean forward and place your head into your hands. This is a critical move.

A common yoga myth is that the head should go fully into the hands so that the hands and fingers make a "cap" around the back of the head. But notice that when you do this, your hands and wrists roll outward. When they do, come up a bit and now try putting some weight on your forearms and hands. It is difficult. In fact, if you straighten your legs and try to put weight down, you will still be able to lift your hands and distal forearms off the floor.

Instead, place your head on the mat a little away from your interlocked fingers, while slowly straightening your knees, roll toward the top of your head so that the back of your head touches your wrists, but your wrists stay turning inward a bit to press the head. You now feel like you could "grab" your head with your top wrists.

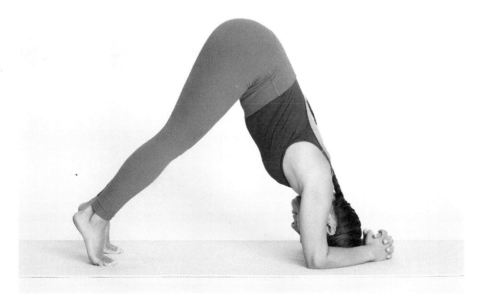

FIGURE 8.13

Your eyes should be parallel to the horizon, your upper wrists pushing your head firmly, and the hands turning slightly toward your head with your fingers firmly interlocked but relaxed. Push your forearms into the floor, lift your shoulders, and then straighten your legs. This position is often called Half Headstand. Remember to breathe and to imagine spreading your shoulders apart while keeping your forearms hugging the sides of your head. After several breaths, come down and repeat one more time.

To continue learning the full Headstand, please contact an experienced teacher who can guide you slowly and well on how to safely learn the full pose at the wall.

MAIN POINTS TO REMEMBER FROM THIS CHAPTER

→ Inversions do not bring more blood or oxygen to the brain.

→ Tradition teaches that inversions have a strong but subtle energetic effect on all aspects of our being.

→ Your upper extremity and your neck are not normally weight-bearing structures, so you need to pay extra attention and use caution when practicing inversions.

→ There are both simpler and more complex inversions, so it is likely that most students can find an inversion they enjoy and that can be practiced safely.

→ Inversions are best when learned from an experienced yoga teacher who can offer individual instructions to each student according to the student's ability and health.

Attentive Practice

Inversions can be dramatic and even fun poses to practice. However, they definitely require balance, strong focus, and careful attention to the demands they make on our hands, wrists, shoulders, and neck. Please make sure that you carefully read the "Cautions" listed below and that if you wish to learn the inversions from category 2, you only do so under the guidance of an experienced yoga teacher.

Remember to take your time. Learn inversions in stages. Look back at chapter 2 and read the instructions for Shoulder Stand at the wall. Notice how it slowly takes you into the pose. This is the key to learning and enjoying inversions: slow and steady.

CAUTIONS

Begin with practicing category 1 poses, but please avoid Headstand, Shoulder Stand, and Handstand if one or more of the following is true:

- You are menstruating or are pregnant.
- It has been less than twelve weeks since you gave birth. (Note that even after twelve weeks, it's a good idea to attain the consent of your medical professional.)
- You have never been taught these poses by an experienced yoga teacher.
- You have GERD (gastroesophageal reflux disease, sometimes called acid reflux disease).
- You have had recent surgery. (Have your medical professional clear you to invert).
- You have a detached retina or glaucoma.
- You have untreated or treated high blood pressure. (Practice only poses from category 1 and show them to your medical professional first for an opinion).
- You are recovering from whiplash or have compromised discs in your neck, and/or any numbness, tingling, or radiating pain in your neck, arm, forearm, wrist, or hand.
- You suffer from arthritis in your neck.
- You are uneasy to try them for any reason.
- You have never practiced yoga asana before. (Please learn the category 2 inversions directly from a teacher in a class before trying them at home.)
- You can't hold Side Plank Pose on your forearm (see figure 7.10 on page 127) with perfect form and steady breath for ninety seconds.

PROPS NEEDED

- Nonslip yoga mat
- Two yoga blocks
- Yoga blanket
- Clear, flat wall surface
- Sturdy chair (optional)

Standing Forward Bend

UTTANASANA

This is a category 1 inversion. In the completed pose, your head will be below your heart. If you have been away from your practice for a while, this is a very simple and natural movement that will get you started on the path to practicing category 2 inversions again.

It is an excellent pose to teach at the beginning of most yoga asana classes, as well as using it at the beginning of your own home practice because it really quiets the mind and brings the focus inward like all other inversions do. As an instructor with many years of teaching behind me, I can testify that Standing Forward Bend is a quick way to get your chatty class to stop talking and be present. It will grab your students' attention quickly and set the stage for the rest of the practice period.

To practice, stand on your yoga mat and separate your feet about ten inches apart. Place a block just in front of each foot. You will be able to use these to support your hands and arms, depending on how far down you go. Make sure the outside borders of your feet are exactly in line with the borders of your mat. Notice that you may feel as if you are internally rotating your thighs or standing in a more pigeon-toed stance. Actually, when you stand with the outer borders of your feet exactly parallel to the border of your mat, you are in a neutral rotation of the hip joint.

You have probably been lining up the inside or arch side of your feet with each other. That alignment choice will actually produce an external rotation of the hip joints. External rotation of the hip joints makes it more difficult to move into deep hip flexion.

Now place your hands on your side hips and inhale. As you exhale, come down into the pose. Remember to continue to exhale softly and evenly as you move downward. It is most important that you keep your chin and your head slightly dropped, and your neck in its normal curve.

Many students have been taught to arch the neck when coming into this pose. You may remember the discussion of the sympathetic curves of the vertebral column that we discussed earlier on page 10. Because of the effect of the sympathetic curves when you arch your neck, you arch your lumbar at the same time.

I do not agree with the yoga myth of arching the neck while coming down into Standing Forward Bend for two reasons. First, arching the neck and thus the lumbar spine actually shortens the back of the vertebral column. Arching your neck is not the way to keep the column long.

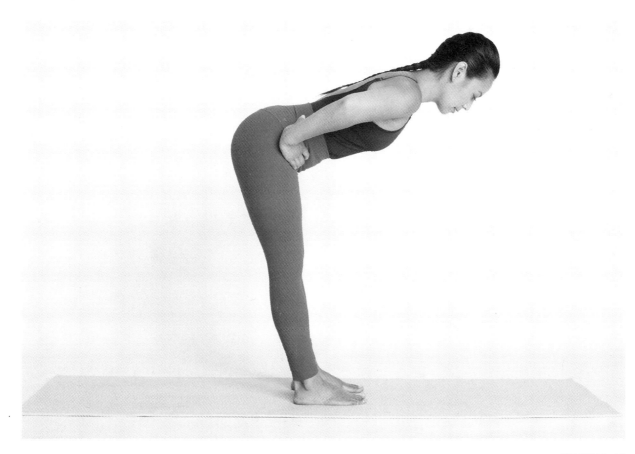

FIGURE 8.14

The vertebral column is the longest when it is in the normal curves. This is anatomical reality. Come down in your normal curves. When you do, you will feel the automatic stabilization of your abdominal muscles in just the right amount.

Second, if you arch your column, you put the abdominals at a mechanical disadvantage, and they cannot support or stabilize your spinal column or abdominal organs very well against the force of gravity pulling down on the trunk as you descend. This is especially true when you are at the point in the movement where the trunk is exactly parallel to the floor. You will also notice that the abdominals automatically contract and gently flex the lumbar spine once you are past 90° of hip flexion. This is normal movement.

By maintaining the lumber curve in neutral, you enable the abdominal muscles to help you the most. If you flex or round all the curves, there is a tremendous amount of weight placed on the lumbar intervertebral discs, hundreds of pounds of force, in fact. If you arch the spinal column, beginning with the cervical spine, it will be harder for your abdominal muscles to support the abdominal organs as well as the column itself in a healthy way.

When you come down into the pose, do not move too slowly; rather, move at a moderate speed. Make sure that you are pulling up on your front thigh

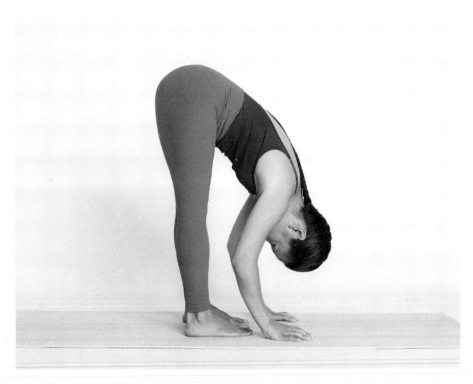

FIGURE 8.15

muscles and not pushing backward on your knees. The backward emphasis at the knees can hyperextend your knees. Place your fingertips lightly on the floor in front of you or on the outer sides of your feet, and breathe. You can also use the two yoga blocks to support your fingers. If you need to, you can put one block on top of the other and place them in front of you to rest on.

Once you have come down into the pose, check and make sure your tibias are exactly vertical. It is necessary to move your pelvis backward in the process of coming down into the pose in order to accommodate gravity; however, once you are down and stable, make sure you are not putting the weight just on your heels but rather on the entire back third of your foot where the ankle joint is.

Make sure you are allowing your head to hang down in a totally relaxed manner. Keep breathing. Do not bend the knees. It is more advantageous to raise the support under your hands and keep the knees straight than to bend the knees to satisfy the ego's desire to touch the floor. Remember, the safest way to practice yoga asana is to prioritize alignment over range.

If at all possible, have your teacher or friend tell you if your sacrum is slanting forward and down in the pose. Another way to say this is that your tailbone should be the highest part of the pose. This means you have created the pose by moving your pelvis over your hip joints. This action will not only

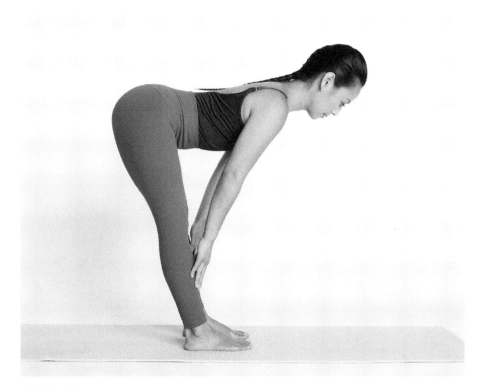

FIGURE 8.16

stretch your hamstring muscles in the back of your thigh, it will also protect your lower back.

To come up and out of the pose, first make sure you are on the tips of your fingers. As you come up, remember to keep your vertebral column in its natural curves again. Place your hands on the front of your legs and come up with a big inhalation.

Stand still for a moment to make sure you are not feeling dizzy. Try the pose once more, this time perhaps varying the width of the feet. If you are on the tighter side, widen the feet. If you are looser, narrow your feet. You will notice that if you make this slight change, the second time you take Standing Forward Bend will be as fresh in sensation as it was the first time.

Here is a technique that can help you get the feeling of moving the pelvis over the head of your femurs when you bend forward in Standing Forward Bend. Take your mat to the wall and place the short end of the mat so that it is touching the wall.

Now stand with your back facing the wall. Open your feet twelve to fourteen inches apart and about fourteen to

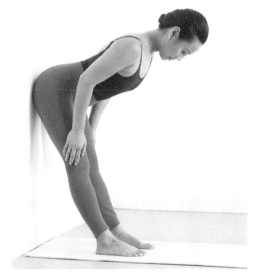

FIGURE 8.17

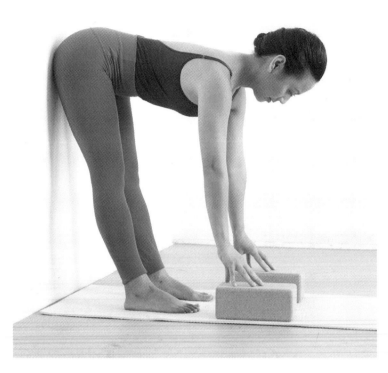

FIGURE 8.18

sixteen inches away from the wall. Slightly move backward so that you are leaning on the wall, and you feel your ischial tuberosities and your coccyx, or tailbone, firmly pressing against the wall.

Exhaling, drop your chin and bend forward while carefully maintaining your normal spinal curves as discussed above. The idea of this technique is to notice how the sitting bones are moving up the wall slowly as you bend. This means you are bending from the hip joints.

The constant even pressure of your sitting bones on the wall indicates that your forward bend is truly coming from the pelvis moving over the heads of your femurs and not from the flexing, or rounding, of your spine, a position that is stressful for the lower back especially. When your sitting bones stop moving, there is instant and clear feedback that the forward bend is not being created by the release of the hamstrings and other posterior leg muscles but by the spinal column.

Stop bending when this happens. Now you know exactly how much of your forward bend is a true forward bend and how much is "fake" because it is coming from your back rather than your pelvis. Next time you practice Standing Forward Bend, you may want to support your hands on blocks or even lean on a stable chair, and go no farther than is appropriate and safe for you.

As you come up, inhale and press your tailbone down the wall. Your arms stay down by your sides and your spinal column stays in neutral. Your abdominals are slightly working, but you still maintain a normal arch in your lower back. Once you are up, take a couple of breaths before practicing your next pose.

Wide-Legged Forward Bend

PRASARITA PADOTTANASANA

This is another category 1 inversion. Step on your mat and spread your feet about four-and-half feet apart. Feel free to experiment with this distance. Make sure the outside borders of your feet are exactly parallel to the border of your mat.

Put your hands on the tops of your thighs as shown in figure 8.19. Drop your head to bring your neck into alignment with the rest of your vertebral column, and keeping your normal curves intact, exhale and bend slowly forward. Be sure to keep your knees completely straight and the kneecaps facing forward.

Now place your fingertips on the floor so that your hands are shoulder width apart. Keep your elbows straight. Check and make sure that you have not pushed your pelvis back as you have come down. The outside of your hip joints should be exactly in line with the outside of your anklebones, other-wise you may inadvertently be hyperextending your knee joints. If it is easy for you, you may place your hands lightly on the outside of your ankles. Be sure to release your head completely and let it hang down.

Keep your breath soft and moving. Make sure that your pelvis is tipped well forward as in the previous pose. When you are ready to come up, place your fingertips on the floor directly under your shoulders with your elbows straight, and hold for a breath. Then place your hands back on your top thighs as previously instructed.

To come up, inhale and pull down to the heels using the muscles in the back of your legs, especially the hamstrings, and keep your lower front ribs

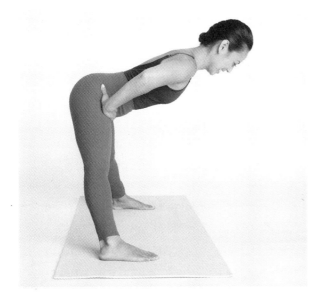

FIGURE 8.19

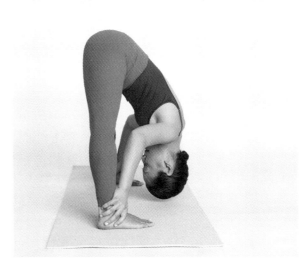

FIGURE 8.20

from pushing forward. You want just the normal arch in your back as you come up. You will feel your abdominal muscles slightly engaging as you lift.

But this action is totally natural, and you do not have to *make* it happen. If you do consciously pull your abdomen in, you will likely overdo this contraction, and the net result will be that you come up with a rounded back, a position that is not healthy for the lower back and the discs there. When you are vertical, take a couple of breaths and repeat the pose again. Both of these category 1 inversions take the head lower than the heart in a way that is generally accessible to most healthy people.

———

The next section of this chapter gives instructions for practicing with category 2 inversions. These poses are much more difficult, requiring a much higher level of body awareness, greater strength and flexibility, and a more sensitive balancing ability.

Honestly, I felt ambivalent about including these poses in this chapter at all, because in my opinion, they should never be learned from a book. We should all learn these poses directly from an experienced teacher who is able to discern if and when we are able to begin these poses, and how the poses might be adapted to each individual student at every stage of learning any of the category 2 inversions.

However, what convinced me to include these poses was what I have observed in many different teaching environments since I began teaching in 1971. These poses have great potential for health and increased self-reflection, but I noticed frequently when I would travel to teach that many students seemed to be ill-trained in the techniques of inversions. Since the advent of the internet, I have noticed that many of the yoga myths about these inversions have been propagated even more widely.

So I decided to include some category 2 inversions here, thinking that I might be able to help some people avoid creating risky habits at the very least and perhaps even prevent injury. I earnestly hope that the readers who practice from my instructions given here are already fully prepared for this practice.

Before you try any category 2 poses, carefully re-read the "Cautions" section above. If in doubt about whether to try these poses, don't.

Do not try these poses for the first time from this book. Seek out an experienced teacher first to teach you well and help you with your first attempts. My fervent wish is that you take care of yourself as you practice category 2 inversions and that you do not let your ambition overcome your innate sagacity or your commonsense awareness of how to take care of yourself. That said, we begin.

Half Handstand at the Wall

ARDHA ADHO MUKHA VRKSASANA

First review the discussion about hand placement offered earlier in this chapter. It is extremely important to pay careful attention to the placement of your hands. They should be at shoulder width apart in this pose and in the next.

What exactly is shoulder width? A widely held yoga myth is that shoulder width is the placement of the hands so that the centers of the palms are in line with the socket of the shoulder joint. But try this: Place your mat near a wall, with the short end touching the wall. Sit on your mat with your back to the wall and lift both arms up to 90° of flexion so that your arms are parallel to the floor.

Notice your collarbones. Do they have a natural width? It is likely that if you place your palms in line with your shoulder joints as is often taught, you will observe easily that your collarbones will not have their natural shape. They will feel squashed. Reach up with one hand and touch your opposite collarbone to see what I mean. Keep this position and imagine that you are pushing a heavy boulder away from you. It probably does not feel like a strong action.

Now widen your arms a bit until you find the exact alignment where your collarbones have their own natural space and shape. This will likely be wider than you thought at first. When you moved your arms outward a bit, did you notice your shoulder blades changed position, perhaps dropping down a bit and widening?

Again, imagine you are pushing a heavy boulder away from you. I am guessing that this time you felt more stability around your shoulder blades and your abdominal muscles spontaneously contracting. You already know why they contracted even though they are not shoulder muscles. As you learned in chapter 7, it is because the abdominals are important, powerful and, in fact, critical trunk stabilizers. When you are pushing a boulder or holding up your body weight against the force of gravity, you need the abdominals to be doing their job stabilizing.

Now come down on all fours with your head facing away from the wall. Once you have placed your hands well on the floor, keep your head up and, starting with your right foot, begin to walk your feet up the wall. It will no doubt take several tries to find the exact distance from the wall from which you want to begin. Try a slightly different distance several times if need be.

Always walk up the wall on your toes and on the whole surface of the balls of your feet and always keep your hands under and slightly wider than your shoulders, your elbows straight, and your head up. There are extensor reflexes in your nervous system that tend to make your limbs extend when your neck is

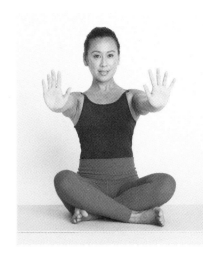

FIGURE 8.21

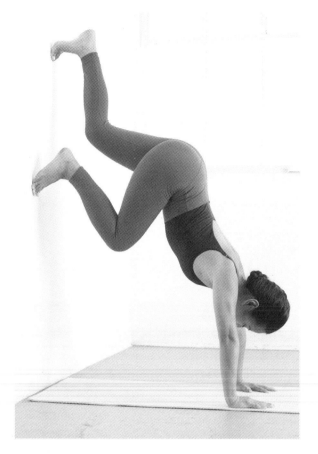

FIGURE 8.22

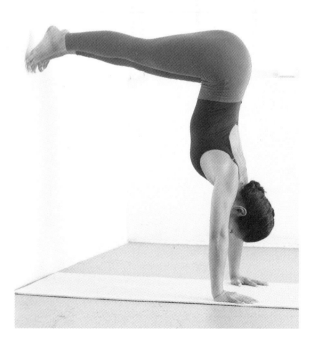

FIGURE 8.23

in extension. Use this reflex to help you keep your elbows absolutely straight by keeping the head a little up and not completely hanging down.

It is perfectly fine—in fact I encourage you—to only walk a little way up the wall as you are learning the pose. Some students practice this pose at home by putting their yoga mat at the bottom of a sturdy staircase. So instead of walking up the wall, they walk up two or three steps backward to get the feeling of Half Handstand and the sensation of weight on their hands, arms, and shoulders.

As you gain strength and confidence, you can walk up to a 90° angle, but still keep your heels away from the wall a bit and the balls of your feet and toes on the wall. This allows you a little space to adjust your body either away from the wall or toward it an inch or two while you are in the pose so you don't have to come down and start over for a small adjustment. You will feel more dynamic in the pose with this little bit of freedom.

There is what I believe to be a yoga myth swirling around that your feet need to be flat on the wall. I find this unnecessary and in fact a hindrance to creating a certain lightness and ease in the pose. But more importantly, I find it actually causes students to feel more weight on their wrists and hands.

Remember, the action is to push yourself upward in the pose, not to push your chest horizontally toward the wall, thus arching your back. Create your normal curves. Breathe easily and stay ten seconds at first. Gradually build up more time as you understand and enjoy the pose more.

Come down by putting your feet on the floor one at a time. Rest a bit and repeat the pose. This time begin by stepping the left foot up first. Half Handstand is stimulating and centering at the same time and is best practiced at the beginning of a session, perhaps following Downward-Facing Dog Pose in your sequence.

Handstand

ADHO MUKHA VRKSASANA

It would be better to learn this pose with a teacher, but once you are confident you understand the way to proceed, begin as you did in the previous pose by putting the short end of your yoga mat against the wall.

Start with your hands facing the wall. Then place your hands on the mat, slightly wider than your shoulders, and create an arch in your hand by pulling the pads of your fingers inward a little to cause the muscles of the palms to engage. This will not only afford stability to your hands and wrists; it will also contribute to your ability to balance away from the wall. If this does not sound familiar, please review the discussion on weight-bearing hand placement in this chapter under "Your Anatomy in Action."

Now put your right leg forward about halfway to the wall, and stand on the ball of your foot.

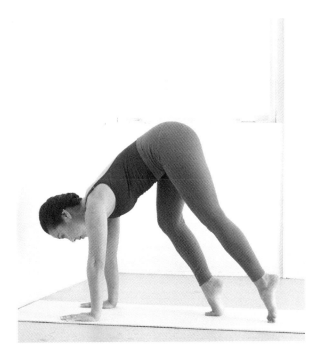

FIGURE 8.24

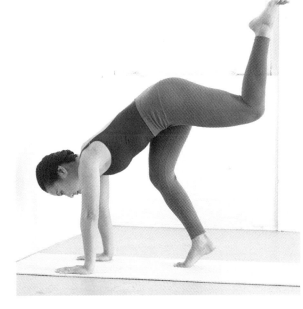

FIGURE 8.25

Shift your weight forward so your shoulders are directly over your hands. This is critical. You do not want your shoulders too far back because not only will you be taking your trunk up as you kick up, you will be moving it horizontally toward the wall. It is much easier to master this pose it you keep your weight well forward; thus, as much of your trunk as possible is forward. Do not collapse into the shoulder joints but continually lift up and "out" of them.

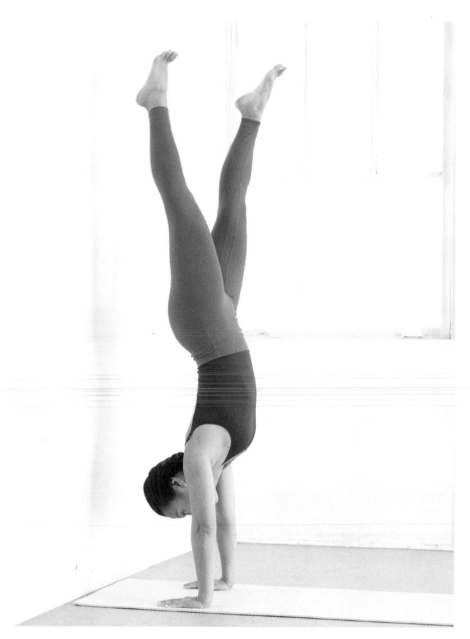

FIGURE 8.26

Keep your head up the whole time. This is very important to help you keep your elbows straight. Your right leg is your "push leg" and your left leg, which is back, is your "swing leg." Most people think it is the swing leg that gets you up, but it is actually the push leg. Most of the work of getting up comes from the right leg now.

Come up onto the ball of your right foot and lift your pelvis as high as you can and toward the wall without losing the vertical position of your arms. Remember, while the legs are propelling you upward, it is easier to get up if you focus on moving your pelvis instead. All you really have to do is to get your pelvis over, or almost over, your shoulders, and your legs will follow. Keep your head up and elbows straight at all times.

Inhale, and with an exhalation, push very strongly with your right foot and ankle. Push firmly to straighten your right knee by using your strong thigh muscles. As this starts to happen, swing your right leg up to join your left, which has already gone most of the way up. However, the action of the right leg should not happen too soon. The left leg must be about two-thirds of the way up before the right leg begins to swing up.

When you are learning the pose, let both heels touch the wall. Rotate your legs inward so the balls of the feet are touching and the heels are slightly apart, and lift up from the inner thigh, stretching up from your inner groin to your inner anklebone. Keep breathing and lift up and out of your shoulders.

Continue to keep your head up. When you have become very familiar with and confident in the pose, you can drop the head once you are up, but please do not try dropping your head until then. It is much safer to keep the head up.

Come down by bringing the right, then left leg down to the floor. You may want to rest in Standing Forward Bend for a few breaths before repeating. I always think it is better to repeat poses at least twice so that what you learned the first time can be impressed upon the nervous system and body memory again.

When going up with the left leg first feels like second nature, then switch to learning to come up with the right leg first. That will bring you back to the lovely state of "beginner's mind" and help you remain humble. If you are a teacher, you will have students who prefer the left leg first. It will help you teach them if you understand from your body, not just your mind, how to come up with either leg first.

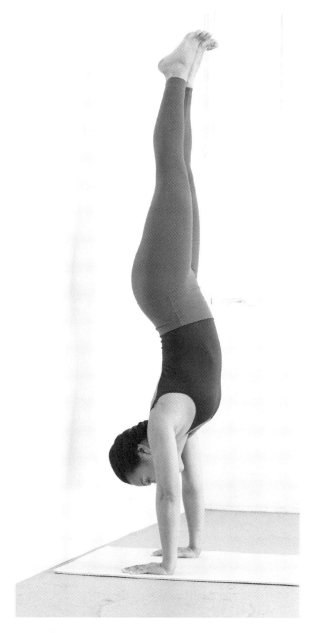

FIGURE 8.27

Elbow Stand

PINCHA MAYURASANA

Many students find this pose more difficult than Handstand because there is more of a challenge to the flexibility of the shoulders and the thoracic spine, or the upper back. I would suggest that you try coming up into the pose the first few times with the help of an experienced teacher.

To begin, spread out your yoga mat near the wall, with the short end of the mat against the wall, and get down on all fours. Place your forearms down on the floor in pronation as you have been instructed in the "Your Anatomy in Action" section of this chapter, on page 139. Make sure that your ulna bones are on the outside of your forearm and that the flesh of your forearm is on the inside. When you do this, you feel the ulna bone pressing the floor evenly and firmly on the outside of your arm.

Make sure that the centers of your palms are in line with your elbows and that your forearms are exactly parallel to each other. Resist the urge to move your elbows out to the side and let your hands move inward. You may enjoy placing a yoga block or two between your thumbs and index fingers to keep the alignment of your forearms pristine. Remember, you want to maintain the normal length of your collarbones as well. So make sure this hand placement is maintained.

If you are ready, straighten your legs and stand on the balls of your feet without disturbing your arms and hands. Make sure that your pelvis is lifted up. To come up, lift up your head and at the same time move your rib cage toward the center of the room. Push your chin out and up.

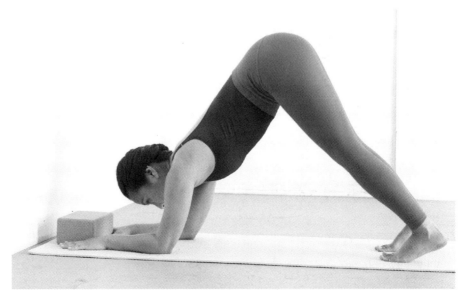

FIGURE 8.28

What is required here is a lot of extension or backbending in your thoracic spine. Thus by lifting your head strongly and moving your rib cage toward the center of the room, you will facilitate backbending throughout the spine.

One of the most important things to remember in the process of kicking up is to move the upper back toward the center of the room while simultaneously holding the shoulders still. Many students start well, but when they kick up their shoulders tend to collapse forward. Push backward with your forearms. All you really need to do is to move your pelvis over your rib cage and the legs will follow. Put your focus on stabilizing the shoulders, arching your thoracic spine and neck, and moving the pelvis over the shoulders, and you will have it.

Now kick up with one leg like you did in Handstand. The right leg is the push leg; most people push with their right foot, so put that foot a little closer to the wall. Keep the pelvis as high as you can. The left leg will be the swing leg and will start the upward movement. Be sure to exhale as you go up. Let your heels lightly hit the wall. Keep breathing.

If you want to learn to balance a few inches away from the wall, put your focus just above your pubic bone halfway to the navel. Pull in here so your legs will move slightly away from the wall and into a vertical position. (See figure 8.6 for the completed pose.)

Remember to keep your head up. Hold the pose, either at the wall or as a balance, for five breaths, then come down one leg at a time. Rest and repeat. As you become adept at this pose, try to learn to practice it by taking your other leg up first.

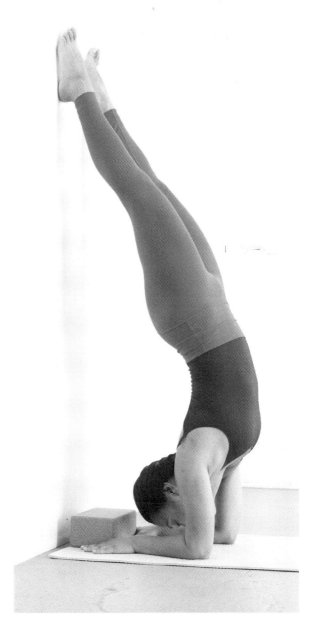

FIGURE 8.29

Half-Supported Headstand

ARDHA SALAMBA SIRSASANA

This beginning practice is designed to help you strengthen muscles that will help you stay in Headstand, as well as mobilize your shoulders and upper back to create flexibility and awareness there. I have taught this variation on its own in my experienced beginner classes because it is useful in and of itself. It can also be taught right before full Headstand.

Spread out your mat and get down on all fours. Now place your elbows down first, then stretch out your forearms and interlock your fingers as was explained in the section above called "Your Anatomy in Action."

Once your forearms are well connected to the floor all along the ulnas, and your fingers are interlocked as instructed earlier on page 141, inhale, then exhale and straighten your legs. Lift your head up. Always remember to keep breathing in every pose. The breath is not only your focal point, it is also a gauge of how much you are exerting. Now inhale, then exhale as you lift up and back into an inverted V.

Now begin to move forward over your forearms and hands, coming as close to a horizontal position as you can.

Once there, lift backward to return to the inverted V position. Keep going back and forth between the two positions several times. You may find that you want to open your legs a bit or walk them forward or backward. The more forward your legs are, the more challenging this movement is; the farther back your legs are, the easier it is.

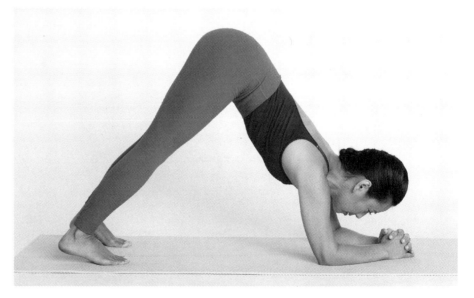

FIGURE 8.30

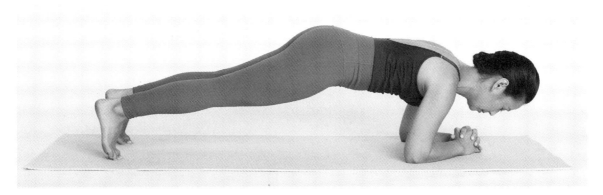

FIGURE 8.31

Keep your wrists vertical or slightly turned in and maintain firm contact on the mat with your ulna bones. Notice how your upper back is moving, how much your shoulder muscles are working, and how your abdominal muscles are naturally engaged as stabilizers. That is why this pose is a great preparation for Headstand, as well as for Elbow Stand. It helps you gain the flexibility and strength necessary for these poses.

After several repetitions, come down and rest. Now unlace your fingers and interlock them in the other direction. To understand what I mean, interlock your fingers in front of your face in the way that feels the most natural to you. For me, it is a position in which my left thumb is on top of my right thumb, my left index finger is on top of my right index finger, my left middle finger is on top of my right middle finger, and so on. Now open your hands, separate them a couple of inches, then interlace them again so that whichever thumb and fingers were on top of their "mates" before are now on the bottom. In my case, my left thumb and all of my left fingers are now beneath their right-hand mates.

Once you have interlocked your fingers in their new position, which will feel, frankly, a little weird, practice Half-Supported Headstand again. Take care to create a firm base before lifting your pelvis and moving forward and back with your breath.

A startling thing I learned when I first did this movement was how much harder it was when I practiced it with my uncommonly used "right thumb on top" position. My muscles were working in a new way. I realized that I had created a habit of using my upper body so as to favor one side of my body. So, I began to practice this pose three times: once on my weaker side, once on my stronger side, and then again on my weaker side. This way of practicing helped me even out my strength from side to side.

Once you are finished, sit back and down on your heels in Child's Pose (see page 182) and rest. Take several long breaths and reflect for a moment. The pauses between the poses are as important to self-awareness as is the time spent in the pose.

Supported Headstand

SALAMBA SIRSASANA

Besides Lotus Pose, Headstand is likely the pose most associated with the practice of yoga asana. Be sure to assess your readiness for this pose with an experienced teacher before you try it. A note to teachers: I almost never introduce this pose to students over the age of fifty-five or so. I give them Half Headstand instead. From the outside, we really have no way as teachers to assess the health of our students' cervical spines. I always err on the side of caution and ease when teaching yoga asana. In my opinion, a professional teacher is creative enough to find other inversions for those who need to work at a different level.

To practice, take your mat to the wall and place it with the short end touching the wall. Now place a firm blanket on the mat to offer some padding to your head. Some students are taught to practice Headstand on a bare floor or on a very thin mat, but I think the top of the head is sensitive and needs a bit of padding. Too thick a blanket, however, will interfere with stability.

Get down on your hands and knees, and place your forearms, hands, and fingers as was instructed on page 141. Remember to slightly separate your little fingers and to turn your top wrist (the radial side) slightly inward.

The next choice is very important. How far into the hands do you place your head? As I mentioned in the "Your Anatomy in Action" section of this

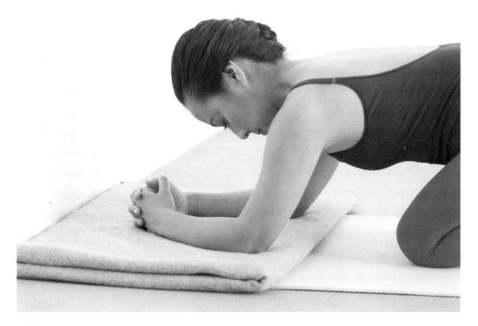

FIGURE 8.32

chapter, another yoga myth I disagree with is to place the head all the way into the hands. In rare instances this works for some people.

Let's try it now. Place your head into your hands very snugly. You will find that doing so causes your wrists to turn outward, and you lose the contact between your upper wrist and your head. Not only that, but you are now no longer moving toward pronation, but instead have supinated your forearms.

Remember our discussion earlier about how pronation and extension go together? Pronating helps you use the triceps muscle in the back of your upper arm, which is the major extensor of the elbow. Using your triceps gives you more leverage and strength to push down with the arms in Headstand. If you put your head deeply into your hands, you will lose the connection of the web spaces between the index fingers, your wrists will roll out, and your forearms will be in supination. This will make it harder for you to effectively use the triceps to push yourself up into the pose.

Now reengage your forearms, hands, and wrists, and place your head against the radial side of your wrists. Your hands are neither completely open nor completely closed. You may even like the sensation of "holding" the sides of your head with your forearms.

Here is a trick about where to place the weight on the top of your head. Begin by placing your weight a little to the front or face side of the exact top of your head. You will be looking slightly down. Thus as you come up into the pose, you will naturally roll toward the top of the head and find your balance

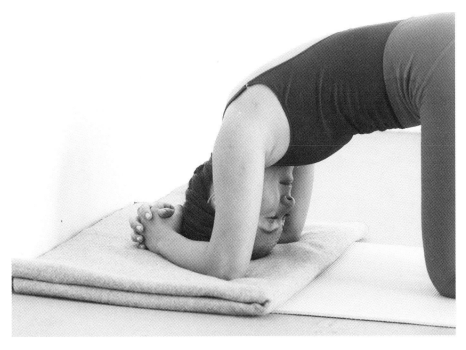

FIGURE 8.33

there. You will be looking straight out into the room. If you go too far and are on the back part of the head, your neck will be too flat; if you are too far forward, your neck will be too arched. Learning this technique may take several tries. Ask your teacher for some help and feedback.

Straighten your legs and walk them in toward your trunk so your knees bend toward your chest. Resist the urge to collapse your shoulders toward the floor. Let your pelvis tip back a bit over your hands so that your feet come off the floor.

Do not attempt to lift with your legs straight. Instead, keep your knees bent. Now kick up with one leg like you did in Handstand. The forward leg is the push leg and the other leg is the swing leg; immediately take your feet to the wall so that your shinbones are parallel to the floor.

Pause here to make sure that your eyes are parallel to the floor and your shoulders are strongly lifted so that your neck is long. The curve in your neck should look like it does when you are standing in Mountain Pose with all your normal curves intact.

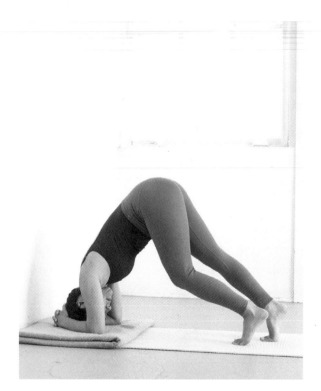 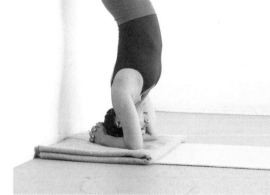

FIGURE 8.34   FIGURE 8.35

If you are new to the pose, stay only for five breaths with your feet on the wall like this, then come down and rest in Child's Pose (see page 182) for several breaths. (Instructions on how to come down safely are given below.) After a few times of practicing this way you can begin to move one leg at a time from the wall to the vertical position. Move slowly as you do this; take your time to find the balance point. I have found that when I focus on my abdomen, at a point midway between the navel and the pubic bone, I find my balance quickly.

Keep the breath easy and natural in the pose. Turn your legs inward so that the balls of the feet touch and the heels separate, and stretch moderately up through the balls of your feet. Constantly monitor the lift of your shoulders and the firm but easy pressure of your wrists at the radius on your head. Look straight out into the center of the room.

Remember that there is no sensation in the neck that is healthy. Feeling some pressure on your head is normal and can be quite pleasant, but if you have any sensation in your neck, come down at once. You may even want to have your neck checked out by a medical professional like a physical therapist, chiropractor, or physiatrist. Do not ignore this sensation.

When you are ready to come down, slowly lower one leg and then the other and immediately sit back on your heels, bring your forehead to the floor, and rest. This is an important step. Headstand has had effects on your cardiovascular system, your organs, your muscles, and your brain. Give yourself a few moments of rest to integrate and appreciate the effects of Headstand before jumping up and moving on.

Unlike most poses, I do not recommend you practice Headstand more than once. It is a strong pose with deep effects, and one Headstand per practice period is sufficient. A lovely sequence is to follow Headstand with Shoulder Stand. They are the yin and yang of inversions and complement each other perfectly. Over time, many students learn to hold these poses for up to five minutes, but that quite depends on the individual.

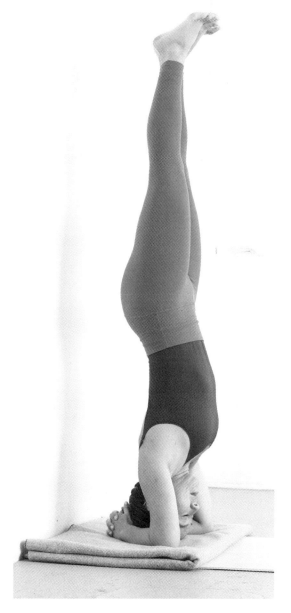

FIGURE 8.36

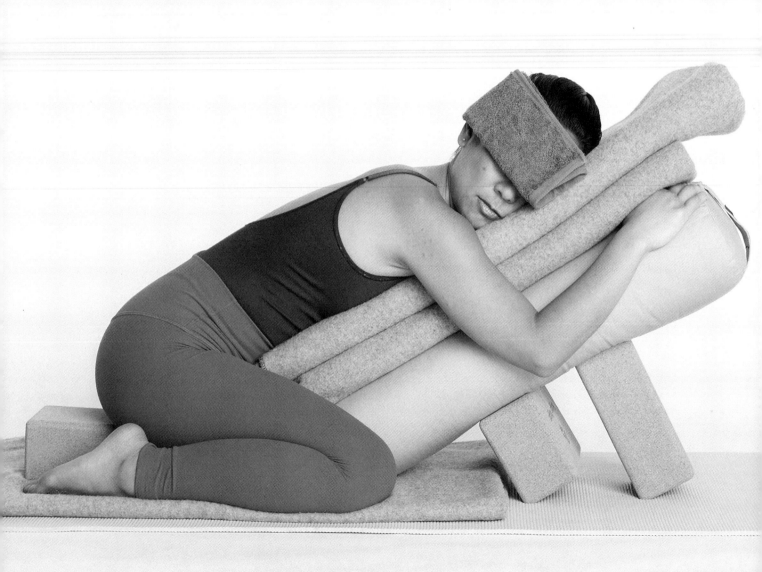

9

Special Times

PRACTICING DURING MENSTRUATION, PREGNANCY, AND MENOPAUSE

Always practice with attention to today's body, not yesterday's.

O N MY FIRST TRIP to study yoga with the Iyengar family at the Ramamani Iyengar Memorial Yoga Institute, in Pune, India, I was eager to expand my practice by working very hard every day in every pose. I had the irrepressible energy of youth and the naïve self-confidence to go with it. I was sure that I could meet any physical or emotional challenge thrown my way.

During the first week, things were rolling along smoothly, but at the beginning of the second week, I got my period. Several long-time students at the Institute informed me that I should participate in the regular class, but because of my period, I needed to practice in a specific part of the back of the room, which was near the open balcony. Furthermore, I was to practice a very particular sequence of poses, mostly consisting of forward bends, some active, some supported. I was to do this particular practice every day for the duration of my period.

I did not like this idea at all. Not only did the balcony open toward the street and allow in the raucous noise of the traffic, it also meant that I was missing the "real yoga practice" of standing poses, handstands, vigorous backbends, and shoulder stands that was going on right in front of me. This vexed me.

My rebellious attitude changed radically when unexpectedly B. K. S. Iyengar himself marched over to me, took off his watch, handed it to me, and then rattled off a series of poses I was to do, saying to hold each one for five minutes on a side. But that was not all. I was to lead all the other women who were practicing this alternative practice with me as well, about eight women in all.

I was to tell them which poses to take, on which side, when to go into the pose, and when to come up. It was a bit like putting the fox in charge of the hen house because I was inwardly rebelling against not practicing with the rest of the class. Suddenly I "owned" the practice in a new way. It was a brilliant move on the part of Mr. Iyengar, and one that I would, over time, come to appreciate greatly.

Under the watchful eye of my teacher, I dared not vary from his instructions. Dutifully I practiced the poses as instructed and was pleasantly pleased to find that they were exactly what I needed that day to balance my energy and draw me into that quiet place inside me, that place where the orchestra of my whole being was playing in perfect sweet harmony. I had learned a lot that day.

When I returned home and continued doing this special practice during my periods, I also wanted to teach other women about this way. As I discussed this approach, I found there were other opinions that differed from mine. So in this chapter, we will discuss the philosophy of practice in relationship to the healthy processes of menstruation, pregnancy, and menopause.

We will explore the yoga myths that swirl round us in the yoga world as we practice asana during these specific healthy normal states. We will consider the asana practice philosophy that traditional teachers from India often espouse for women in these states. And we will compare and contrast this with the philosophy of asana practice espoused by those yoga teachers born and bred into a decidedly feminist Western viewpoint.

Hopefully this open-minded approach will help us each to understand the yoga myths that affect our choices regarding practicing as women and what is right for our own bodies. This self-knowledge is what the entire teachings of yoga are about after all.

Why You Need to Know This

It may seem obvious, but there is more to the practice of yoga than just the physical body. Yoga classes in the West are as varied as one can imagine. Some seem to me to be "exercises with Sanskrit names." On the other end of the spectrum there are asana classes that hardly move and challenge the students at all. There is also everything in between.

What I want to introduce here is the ancient idea of cosmic or universal Prana, the idea that there is energy moving through us that is the life force itself. Prana is similar to "chi," the energy that acupuncturists work with to balance us using needles and herbs. This energy can be strong or weak, blocked or agitated, felt or ignored, but it is nonetheless there in all human beings.

While the study of Prana is a lifetime study, I would like to begin by introducing the five main manifestations, or *pranas vayus* (winds), of Prana in the body:

- Lowercased prana (as distinguished from universal Prana, with a capital P) governs the heart and respiration. It tends to move upward.
- *Apana* controls the abdomen below the navel and all the organs there like the kidneys and genitals. It tends to move toward the feet.
- *Samana* lives between prana and apana and controls digestion and the organs of digestion
- *Udana* controls the head and neck and the eyes, ears, tongue, and nose. It controls the limbs and sensory awareness of the body in general.
- *Vyana* is everywhere and as such controls all the other pranas vayus and our movements.

While there are five main pranas vayus, we will only focus on prana and apana in this chapter in relation to the effects of the poses on women experiencing menstruation, pregnancy, and menopause.

The reason I include these principles of prana and apana in this book on yoga myths is that I believe that we are sometimes not fully aware of the actual power of the poses we practice and teach. We may be aware of how yoga asana can increase flexibility and strength in the muscles, but we are often unaware of the deeper effects that yoga asana, especially inverted poses, can have on us energetically.

To illustrate this point, I would like to share a story with you. Years ago, a woman attended a weekend workshop I was teaching and told me about her recent medical history. What she told me was consistent with the idea that her apana energy was not moving as freely as it should. I suggested a series of poses for her that I felt would stimulate and thus increase her apana energy, as well as encourage it to move as freely and normally as it should and help her periods function normally as a result. She spent all the weekend classes only doing a series of poses that tradition teaches us helps to move apana in a healthy way.

The workshop ended on Sunday, and by Tuesday she emailed me that her condition had completely resolved, as verified by her doctor. Of course, this result just could have been a chance happening. But I have had many of these experiences over decades of teaching.

To be clear, I am not suggesting yoga asana as a cure-all or a substitute for professional medical help, but I do believe that the practice of asana can have profound effects on our health.

Another story I would like to share was told to me by a yoga student who was part of a closely knit meditation community. She would frequently join one- to three-week-long meditation retreats.

She recounted to me that during such retreats, women attendees often would no longer get their period. I am certainly aware that stress, trauma, low body fat, extreme fatigue, excessive air travel, or illness can interfere with women's regular periods, but never a meditation retreat. I once asked a well-known physiologist why this might happen, and he was flummoxed by my question and did not have an answer to offer.

I don't either. But I do know from personal experience, from teaching yoga classes since 1971, and from interaction with other women yoga teachers that a yoga asana practice does have an effect on the menstrual rhythms and functioning of yoga students.

What I am suggesting here is that we explore together the subject of the practice of yoga asana as it relates to women. I ask that you try some of the poses presented later in this chapter. I also ask that you try paying attention to the effect these recommended poses have on you physically, mentally, emotionally, and energetically during the special times we are discussing.

The first question I am raising is this: Why do we believe that all people, regardless of age, condition, or life circumstance, and sometimes women in special states, should all practice exactly the same way? This is the biggest yoga myth of all. I do not practice like I did in my twenties. Each decade of my life has influenced my practice by shaping it into what was exactly right for me at the time. Sometimes I needed challenge, while other times I needed rest. Sometimes I needed a comforting routine, and sometimes I needed to shake up my routine in order to keep my practice fresh.

The point is that each asana should be a question that we ask ourselves every time we practice a pose. Instead, we usually tell the body what to do instead of listening to what the body is telling us. One of the great benefits of menstruation, pregnancy, and menopause is that the innate intelligence of the body can, and often does, take charge during these times.

If we are wise, we will let this happen and thus become more receptive to the phenomenal wisdom of our body. We will hear its whispers and its needs. We will enjoy its changing state and allow ourselves to cultivate contentment with the changing body in which we live.

Your Structure

The female body is a wonder. It can grow a baby in an organ that can expand up to fifty times its pre-pregnant size and then return to that size after the baby is born. The female brain is bathed in natural chemicals that give us the urge to nurture and to connect with others. We can run marathons, direct symphony orchestras, and excel in every type of academics and in all professions.

However, not all women are alike; far from it. But we generally share the same physiological hormones and are affected by them. One interesting fact about women is that we have more nerve connections between the two hemispheres of our brain and can charge along mentally on this super highway of neural connections. Because of this, regrettably, we are superb at multitasking.

Multitasking is the opposite of yoga. Yoga practices are about enabling us to step back from the rampages of our normal thinking brain. Research has shown that multitasking makes us think we are more efficient, but we actually are not. Human brains were designed to do one thing at a time. I suggest we take up a new practice that I like to call "unitasking." Let's try living our yoga by doing one thing at a time. It will reduce stress and perhaps contribute to our lives by reminding us of the beauty of this very moment, as we give ourselves to each unique moment of our lives.

But of course, women are different from men in other ways than just the way our brain connects. One is that women have a different anatomical structure of the pelvis than men. When the tiny matter that will eventually become a human being is just starting to grow in the uterus, unless that matter is acted upon at a specific time during its development by male hormones, it will have a female pelvis, i.e., an obstetric pelvis. This makes sense from Nature's point of view. It means that Nature's default pelvis is female, not male. When in doubt, better to make an obstetric pelvis than not.

Ironically, all anatomy books discuss the male pelvis and how the female pelvis differs from the "standard" male pelvis. It is interesting to note that because the first anatomists were likely men, it was assumed that the male pelvis was the default.

Deep inside this female pelvis are the vagina, uterus, fallopian tubes, and ovaries. According to traditional wisdom, the pelvis is also home to apana energy, the energy that lives below the diaphragm. During menstruation and pregnancy, apana is very high. So, it would make sense during these times to avoid practicing poses like inversions that increase an apana that is already high. Yet often the yoga myth persists that any woman, menstruating or pregnant, can continue to practice exactly as she does when not menstruating or pregnant.

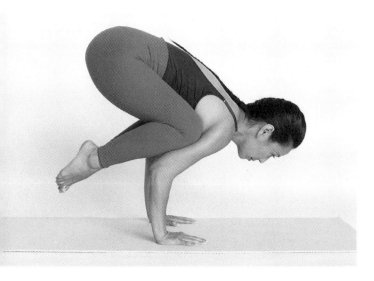

FIGURE 9.1

Furthermore, active poses like standing poses, arm balances like Crow Pose (Bakasana) shown in figure 9.1, along with other arm balances and inversions tend to dampen down apana and fuel prana in the chest.

Backbends can also increase prana, although some supported backbends can be used to increase apana. Too much prana can take a woman out of balance, just like too little apana can.

If women are going to practice yoga asana during all the stages of life, it is important, I believe, that we think not only about the physical aspects of the poses, but also about the energetic aspects. It is important as well that yoga teachers have some understanding of the Prana system and the subtle but powerful effect of the energy that moves through our bodies.

Yet the yoga myth persists that any woman, menstruating or pregnant, can continue to practice any asana with no effect on the function of menstruating or on a pregnancy. If the poses are not affecting us, then why are we doing them?

Your Anatomy in Action

Some of the questions we will answer in this section are: What poses especially act on apana? Which poses could be considered to be "cooling," and which are "heating" or activating to the organs in the female pelvis? How do yoga asana affect the endocrine organs like the ovaries?

The endocrine glands are generally under the power of the pituitary gland at the center of the brain. The pituitary is often called the "master gland" because it helps to regulate all the others. Other endocrine glands include the thyroid and parathyroid, the thymus, the hypothalamus, and the pineal gland, as well as the adrenal glands, the pancreas, and the testes or ovaries.

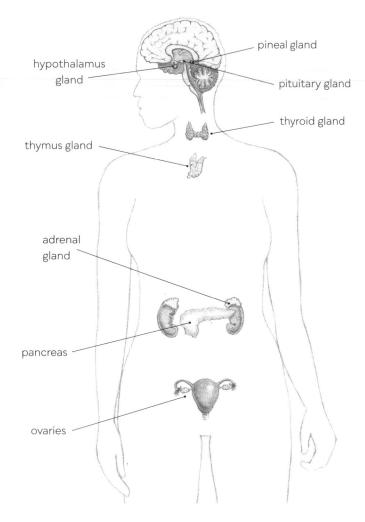

hypothalamus gland

pineal gland

pituitary gland

thyroid gland

thymus gland

adrenal gland

pancreas

ovaries

FIGURE 9.2

The basic principle that I have been teaching in my teacher trainings is this: whatever is open and elevated is stimulated, and whatever is closed and lowered is quieted. Using this idea can be a basic way to start paying attention to the effects of the poses during menstruation, pregnancy, and menopause.

Here is an example. In Supported Bridge Pose, the brain is lower, and the abdomen is not only higher, but also open.

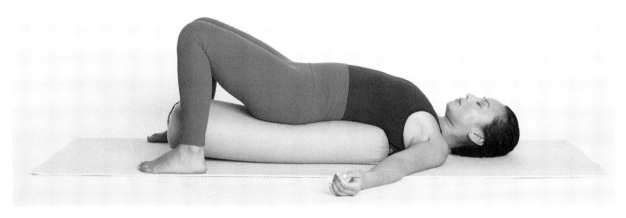

FIGURE 9.3

So this pose would be quieting to the brain and stimulating to the organs of the pelvis like the intestines and the female reproductive organs. I would not give this pose during menstruation because apana is already high, and stimulating it more would create an imbalance. Instead, I would give this pose if someone were constipated or if periods were irregular or if the woman was having trouble getting pregnant.

Another example might be Seated Forward Bend.

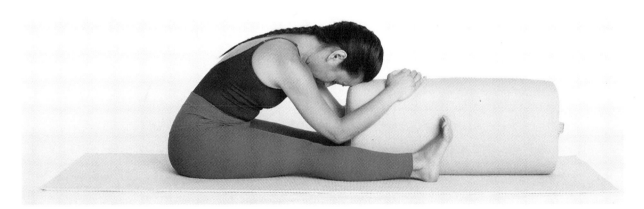

FIGURE 9.4

In this classic forward bend, the pelvis is closed and low, therefore according to our premise, the abdominal organs would be quieted. That is why this pose is useful during menstruation, and with a bolster for support and wider legs, it is also useful during pregnancy when apana is high.

Inversions have an interesting effect on apana. Remember that apana always moves toward the feet. So when you are up in Shoulder Stand, for example, apana now has the freedom to move strongly from the diaphragm toward the pelvic floor. The pelvis is both open and elevated, so apana is stimulated. Therefore, I believe that it is not a good idea to practice this pose during menstruation because it would tend to increase apana too much and thus interfere with the natural state of apana during the period.

Some students who did not follow this guideline found that their period stopped suddenly and then started again, but this time it was too heavy. So instead I suggest poses that reduce the already heightened apana, like forward bends, both active and supported.

After I returned from India where I had had my epiphany regarding practicing during the period, I began to notice that my energy shifted the day before my period. When this happened, I inevitably felt a sense of relief that somehow I had "permission" to take care of myself. I realized that I was having the urge to do a very quiet practice instead of my usual "go go go, hold the poses forever, time my headstand and shoulder stand" approach.

So, I began to practice supported forward bends and a few other quiet poses beginning the day *before* my period actually began. This, I believe, helped me to have an easier experience during my periods. They became predictably regular, slightly shorter, and without cramps. I soon completely let go of the yoga myth that I should not let my period affect my practice. I was happy to let it.

Being pregnant and practicing yoga asana was another revelation. My attachment to the yoga myth that pregnancy did not matter that much when I practiced was lurking in the background of my mind. Luckily my body took over in a big way. On some days, morning sickness was such that I was lucky if I could do Deep Relaxation Pose and some breathing. Other days I was bursting with energy. I felt that my body was the teacher and my mind the student instead of the other way around. As the body as teacher had to be followed, there was no escape. Another yoga asana myth dissolved away.

Pregnancy is another state in which the apana energy is very strong. For this reason, poses like inversions that increase apana are not recommended. But there are other reasons to avoid inversions during pregnancy.

During the first trimester, about thirteen and one-third weeks along, implantation is happening as well as the development of the placenta. In my opinion, this is not a good time to turn upside down. I am glad that there have not been specific studies done on this topic because it would be unethical to do so.

But common sense told me that inversions were not what I really wanted to practice during this time, and I certainly will not teach other women to invert during the first trimester. Please hear this: while some yoga practitioners say they feel fine inverting during the first trimester, no one can really know what is happening inside the pregnant uterus with any certainty in a yoga class. I doubt seriously that women all through history have stood on their head during the first trimester of their pregnancy!

I do not recommend inversions during the second trimester either because the baby's birth position is not yet fixed. I believe that it could be possible that inversions at this state might cause the cord to wrap around the baby. This can also happen when women don't invert, but why borrow trouble? Anecdotally, I have heard of a number of pregnant women who continued inversions, even Handstand, during pregnancy, whose babies were born with the cord wrapped around their neck. This is something to consider.

It is possible to turn a breech baby's position by using a modified inversion done at a specific angle. The mother lies on a "slant board" during certain weeks of pregnancy for a specific amount of time every day. If this has been proven to turn many breech babies, then it logically follows that inverting, and thus changing the pull of gravity on the baby can cause it to turn around. Why invert during pregnancy if you don't need to turn a breech? Perhaps practicing yoga inversions during pregnancy could create a breech presentation where none was present before. Once the pregnancy is over and the postnatal body has returned to normal, then slowly and gradually add inversions back into your practice.

Pregnancy is a healthy normal state, but nonetheless, it is an unusual state. During my first pregnancy, I had an attitude of wanting to prove I wasn't affected in any way by the pregnancy, that I could do physically whatever I had done before, even jogging. I remember that the "nicest" thing I heard from friends was, "You don't look seven months pregnant." I took this as a compliment. But later I was to wonder: what was wrong with looking seven months pregnant anyway?

There is a lot of societal pressure put on the pregnant woman. One example is that others, even strangers, think they have the right to come up and touch the pregnant belly, or offer advice or stories, which usually start with something like, "My sister had the most horrible birth." This is not what pregnant women need. Instead of adding to such pressure, pregnant women need to trust themselves more, rest every day, practice simple poses, and find joy in the present moment. It is unlikely they will find it in Headstand.

The third trimester is not the time for inversions either. Apana is quite high during the third trimester. Inverting could increase it even more. The abdominal muscles, which feel toned and firm to the touch, are actually quite stretched and not as strong as they feel. Just the act of getting up into an inversion like Shoulder Stand may require lying on the back to begin with, which is not a good idea (more on this later), and the act of throwing the legs up into Headstand or Handstand requires abdominal strength that may not be there.

Once the pregnant woman is up in the inversion, now there is the weight of the baby, the placenta, the enlarged uterus, the amniotic fluid, and all the abdominal organs "falling downward" onto the diaphragm. This may make it difficult to breathe. It no doubt increases the intrathoracic pressure.

But even more importantly, it could interfere with the head-down, pre-birth position of the baby. I know this because there is proof that lying a

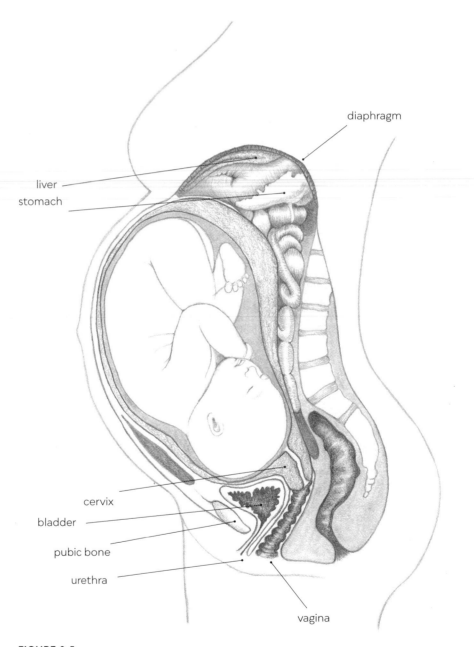

FIGURE 9.5

thirty-two- to thirty-five-week pregnant woman in a very specific supported head-down position can actually encourage the baby to turn to the normal head-down position. If the baby can be stimulated to turn head down by an inversion on purpose, it makes sense that a yoga asana inversion could also stimulate the baby to turn into such a position.

This is interesting evidence of the power of inversions. Personally, I am convinced of two things: first, that inversions are powerful poses, and second, there is really no reason to invert a pregnant woman in yoga class, and lots of reasons not to.

Finally, lying on the back for long periods in a yoga pose is not something I encourage for women after the first trimester of pregnancy. This is because of a physiological process called inferior vena cava syndrome.

The vena cava is the main vein that returns blood from the lower body to the heart. Notice in figure 9.6 how the vein is on the right side of the bodies of the vertebrae. Remember that veins, unlike arterioles and arteries that carry blood from the heart to the body, do not have muscular walls. This means that arterioles and arteries can hold their shape but veins cannot.

Veins can be compressed by pressure. They can also expand to hold more and more blood, especially if the delicate valves are damaged. This is what

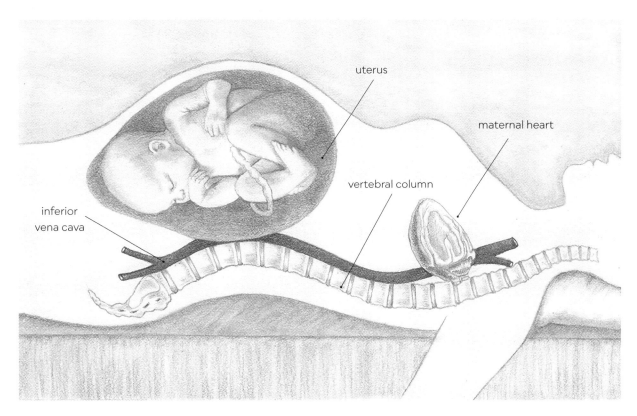

FIGURE 9.6
Inferior vena cava compressed when lying on the back near the end of pregnancy

happens when varicose veins are created. Because arterioles and arteries have a muscular layer, they can contract and relax to move blood in and out. Thus, there is no such thing as varicose arteries.

If a pregnant woman lies on her back for an extended duration, especially at the end of pregnancy, the weight of the baby, enlarged uterus, placenta, and amniotic fluid all fall back onto the vena cava and can interfere with the return of blood to the maternal heart. That means that the maternal cardiac output is reduced, and blood and thus oxygen to the placenta and baby are reduced. The mother may feel like she is going to pass out and the baby may experience some distress from lack of oxygen.

Not all women feel lightheadedness at the end of pregnancy when lying on the back, and some can feel it earlier than others. Perhaps this process of compression can be happening without pregnant women knowing it. Whatever the case may be, why not practice and teach in the safest way to keep mother and baby happy and healthy?

Inferior vena cava syndrome can be avoided simply by elevating the woman's trunk when she is lying down as will be shown in the "Attentive Practice" section below. Pregnant students can also be offered Side-Lying Deep Relaxation Pose when other students are lying on their backs in the class. (For instructions on Side-Lying Deep Relaxation Pose, see my book *Restore and Rebalance: Yoga for Deep Relaxation*, pages 114–19.)

If you teach Side-Lying Deep Relaxation Pose to pregnant women, have them lie on their left side. Look again at figure 9.6. Because the inferior vena cava is slightly to the right, obstetricians usually advise their patients to lie on the left side to avoid compressing the vena cava. I always ask my pregnant students to lie on their left side for this reason. If you are pregnant, you can practice Side-Lying Deep Relaxation Pose this way yourself.

I would like to offer one more caution about inversions, and this concerns the post-partum period. Many dedicated yoginis are eager to invert after the baby is born because they miss their inverted practices. However, after pregnancy there is a vaginal discharge called the lochia that lasts for four to six weeks while the lining of the uterus is healing from the birth of the placenta.

After the lochia has completely stopped, and you feel you are mentally ready to begin inversions again, check with your professional health-care provider to make sure you are physically ready as well. Do not try inversions until at least six weeks after. This can cause the lochia to increase in flow instead of diminish, maybe in part because the inversion has increased apana, which is still high during the early post-partum period. Whenever you do begin inversions again, start slowly and simply with just putting your legs up for a few minutes, or by doing Downward-Facing Dog Pose, and see how your body reacts before moving to more advanced inversions like Headstand.

Finally, the last distinctive stage of a women's life is the stage past the capacity of reproduction: menopause. The female body changes with menopause, just like it changed when puberty began. The changes that accompany menopause can affect the way your body moves in yoga asana.

Notice if you are clinging to the yoga myth that, if you are a woman with a vigorous practice, then your yoga asana practice should remain unchanged during this stage of life. Let your wisdom, gained by years of life and thoughtful yoga asana practice, express itself.

Notice how you may be more drawn to practice *pranayama* (breathing practices), Restorative yoga, and meditation and less drawn to practice the active yoga asana you did before. But maybe some days you will feel more like yourself when you do practice vigorously. My request is that when you are in this stage of life that you listen to yourself with more confidence and trust enough to let yourself "simply be the yoga," both while practicing the poses and in living your life day to day as well. Let the compassion you have developed for yourself shine out on others.

The later years are the perfect time to let your body guide your yoga asana practice more than ever before. Invariably for most women, this guidance will call you to challenge yourself less and feel yourself more, to bow to your inner wisdom.

Whether or not one has become a mother, menopause is an inevitable part of aging. Menopause is defined as the absence of a period for one full year. Many women, however, have symptoms during what is called the perimenopausal years, which can last from five to seven years before the period ceases totally.

Perimenopause usually begins around the midforties, but there is the inevitable range of normal times to begin. Symptoms of perimenopause can include but are not limited to irregular periods, hot flashes, breast tenderness, mood swings, depression, shoulder pain, lessening of libido, fatigue, sleep disturbances, and vaginal dryness. These are directly related to the slow change in a number of hormones that happens with age.

Perimenopause is the perfect time to make your yoga practice very regular and important. Many women in perimenopause have found that supported backbends and supported inversions are the best poses for evening out symptoms.

I suggest you make these types of poses about 50 percent of your practice because they are good for increasing apana, which might be low. If there is a period, though, go back to the type of practice suggested earlier, which reduces apana.

MAIN POINTS TO REMEMBER FROM THIS CHAPTER

→ Yoga asana are more than physical positions, and honoring the expression of Prana in the body is important.

→ Poses that quiet apana during menstruation are very soothing.

→ Inversions are better not practiced during pregnancy.

→ Perimenopause and menopause can be helped by poses that increase apana.

Attentive Practice

There are so many poses that are beneficial for women during menstruation, pregnancy, and the perimenopausal and menopausal years, it was hard to pick just three. Hopefully these three will be of help in your practice and teaching. They have been in mine.

CAUTION

Avoid Child's Pose if you have a knee injury or knee pain. Instead practice Chair Child's Pose, which you can find in my book *Restore and Rebalance*, on pages 28–33.

Make sure the outer legs are well propped in Supported Bound Angle Pose (Supta Baddha Konasana) to prevent any strain to the pubic symphysis or sacroiliac joint of a pregnant woman. The ligaments holding these joints are naturally loosened during pregnancy due to the presence of the hormone relaxin.

Avoid Half Shoulder Stand if one or more of the following is true:

- You are menstruating or are pregnant.
- It has been less than twelve weeks since you gave birth. (Note that even after twelve weeks, it's a good idea to attain the consent of your medical professional.)
- You have GERD.
- You have had recent surgery. (Have your medical professional clear you to invert.)
- You have a detached retina or glaucoma.
- You have untreated high blood pressure.
- You are recovering from whiplash or have compromised discs in your neck, and/or any numbness, tingling, or radiating pain in your neck, arm, forearm, wrist, or hand.
- You suffer from arthritis in your neck.
- You are uneasy to try it for any reason.
- You have never practiced yoga asana before. (Please learn this pose directly from a teacher in a class before trying it at home.)

PROPS NEEDED

- Nonslip yoga mat
- Bolster
- Three yoga blocks
- Up to six yoga blankets
- Bare wall
- Yoga belt
- Eye cover
- Timer

Supported Child's Pose
SALAMBA BALASANA

Here is a pose I recommend to menstruating women. Notice that it is not an inversion, and that the abdomen is closed and low to reduce apana, which is high during menstruation.

Spread out your yoga mat and put a blanket down for padding. Note the fold of the blanket that the model is using in figure 9.7. Starting on your knees, place a yoga block beneath you and sit back on the block, making sure that it is resting on its largest and most stable surface.

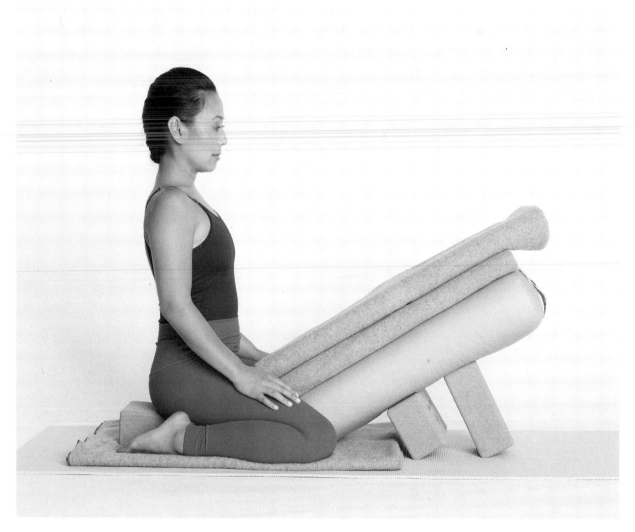

FIGURE 9.7

Place the other two blocks one very tall and one of medium height in front of you, as shown, and place your bolster on top of them, with the short end of the bolster between your legs and as close to your body as you can get it. Make sure the bolster feels steady and the blocks won't tip. Place a folded blanket longways on the bolster, and push the end of the blanket down between your legs. You may decide later that you need another blanket for more height.

Some students like to tightly place a belt all around the belt on the long side of bolster. Make sure the belt is tight. When you take the pose, you can place your hands near the floor and then angle your hands upward, and slide them under the belt. This is an easy and comfortable way to support your arms.

Now lean forward and lie on the bolster so that the blanket(s) presses firmly but pleasantly into your abdomen. Turn your head to one side. You will probably enjoy covering your eyes. Slide your hands and forearms from underneath the belt toward the ceiling so that the belt will hold your arms in a comfortable position. Before you are completely settled, you may want to drape a heavy folded blanket on your back from just below your shoulder blades to cover your whole pelvis. The heavier the blanket is, the better. The weight will feel soothing.

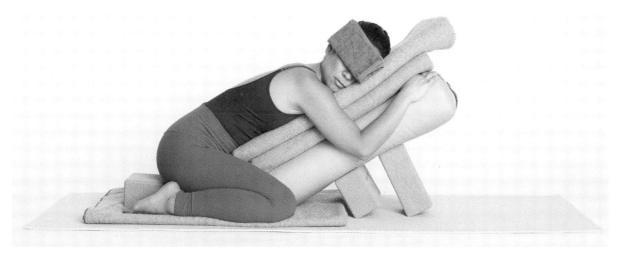

FIGURE 9.8

Hold the pose for one to five minutes. Make sure you turn your head to the opposite side for half of the pose. Breathe into your back body, close your eyes, tuck your chin, and relax.

To come out of the pose, turn the head so your forehead is down on the bolster and take a couple of breaths. Then slip your arms out of the belt and sit up. To come completely out now, lean forward so you are on your hands and knees. Turn your toes under, straighten your knees, and walk backward until all of your weight is on your feet. Inhale as you stand up. This way of coming up will protect your knees.

Here is a variation you can try if you have menstrual cramps. Set your pose up exactly as before, except that you will not need the belt. Once you are seated, and before you bend forward, make fists of your hands.

Place the inside of your wrists on the ASIS. Point each hand diagonally downward toward your pubic bone so as you lean forward, your fist pushes strongly into the lower abdomen right above your pubic bone. When you lie down on the bolster, make sure you drop your elbows down and relax your shoulder area.

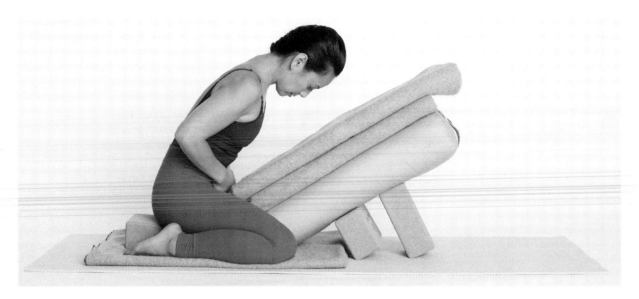

FIGURE 9.9

There should be a lot of pressure in your lower abdomen, and it should feel good. Many students have reported to me that this counterpressure against the uterus can reduce or even stop menstrual cramps. Hold the pose for five minutes as instructed above. Remember to breathe into your back body. Come up by turning your face downward and use your hands to help you sit up. Once again, stand up by taking the weight back on your feet, walking backward, and inhaling as you straighten up.

Supported Bound Angle
SUPTA BADDHA KONASANA

Pregnant women love this pose because it allows them to open and yet to be held and surrender at the same time. Unfold your yoga mat and gather your props.

Arrange your bolster and blocks as is instructed for Child's Pose, but this time you will use two bolsters. Some people find this simpler and more stable. But if you only have one bolster, then use the blocks as shown in figure 9.10. Make sure your bolsters are placed in such a way that they support your back firmly and in a very stable manner. Now lay a long-fold blanket on your top bolster.

Gather your other props closer and sit at the end of your bolster with the soles of your feet together. Now lean forward and walk your pelvis backward; the goal here is to make sure your lower back body is firmly pressed against the bolster all the way from the floor upward. If there is a gap at this area, you will sag down, and the chest will not be open. Do not let the lower back be unsupported.

Once you have this position, roll two blankets up so that they are quite thick and

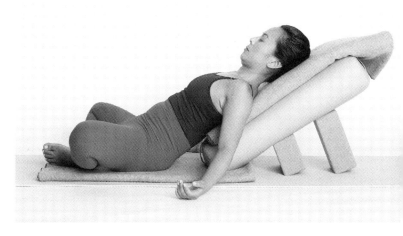

FIGURE 9.10

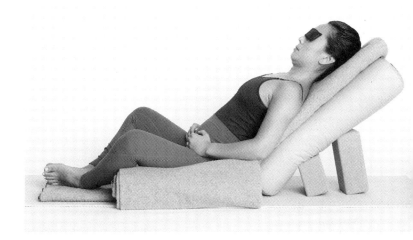

FIGURE 9.11

place them deeply into the outer hip joint. Your intention here is not to support the *knees*, but the *femurs* at their root at the hip joint. Use this support even if you are flexible enough to easily rest your thighs on the floor. Do this *especially* if you are flexible.

If you are not very flexible, you will definitely need support to feel comfortable for the twenty minutes I would like you to stay in this pose in order to reap its full benefits. But if you are flexible, practicing this pose for twenty minutes with the legs open and with the effects of pregnancy hormones in your body like relaxin can overstretch the ligaments of the sacroiliac joint, as mentioned in chapter 3, page 45. Remember that the sacroiliac joint is a joint of stability, not mobility. The job of ligaments is to hold bone to bone, and if the ligaments are too stretched, they cannot do this. No time is a good time to overstretch ligaments, but pregnancy is the most important time not to. Once overstretched, ligaments do not have the structural ability to go all the way back to a normal length.

Once your legs are supported and settled, use either blocks or two more rolled blankets to support your elbows. Place your hands on your top thighs to check whether they are comfortable, and whether your hands are higher than your elbows. This position of "hand higher" is important because it offers more comfort and stability to the shoulder joint. If your arms hang down, this tractions the shoulder joint too much.

Now add some support under your neck if you wish. You may want to roll the end of the long blanket on the bolster well under your neck. Make sure you support from the seventh cervical–first thoracic area, the "big bump" you feel where your neck becomes trunk. Do not just put a roll under your neck. (More detailed information on creating neck support can be found in chapter 11, page 225.) But make sure that your chin is lower than your forehead. This will help your brain quiet.

Be sure to turn off the ringer on your phone, but do set a timer for twenty minutes at least. Actually, I like to set mine for twenty-two minutes or so, which gives me a couple of minutes to get finally settled before my "official" twenty minutes begins. I have actually practiced this pose for a full hour. But twenty minutes is the amount of time that really allows the nervous system to switch into and settle into relaxation mode.

Now put on your eye cover and cover up your whole body with a blanket. Begin to let yourself sink into the support of the props. The idea is not to be feeling a stretch, but rather feeling a "floaty" kind of ease. Begin to watch your breath rise and fall like a soft ocean swell rises and drops. You may enjoy taking a series of five to ten soft, long, full breaths through your nose. (More instruction on specific breathing can be found in the "Why You Need to Know This" section of chapter 10.)

Allow yourself to be sucked inward, away from the outermost boundaries of your body, slowly curling inward with your awareness, like a lazy cat gratefully curls up in front of a warm fire. Consciously move your focus beneath your thoughts. Remain in stillness, silence, and ease. If you wish, send welcoming and soothing energy to the baby growing inside you.

When your timer goes off, be slow to move out of the pose. First bring your knees together, and carefully roll to the left and off the props to lie on your left side for a while. When you are ready, use your hands and arms to help you sit up. Move slowly as you stand up and continue with your day.

Legs-Up-the-Wall Pose

VIPARITA KARANI

VK, as it is often called in yoga classes, is a supported inversion that increases apana, opens the chest, and puts the brain lower than the heart, which actually causes a change in brain waves and is often suggested for the topsy-turvy symptoms of perimenopause, as well as during the latter years of a woman's life. Remember to skip this pose if you are menstruating.

Start by placing the short end of your mat against the wall. Place a block between the wall and your bolster. Fold a blanket in a long-fold shape and

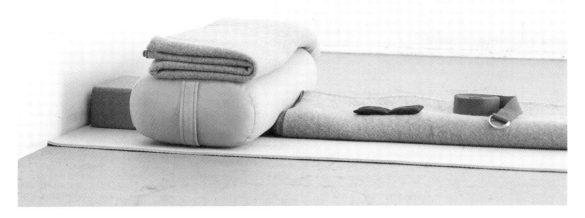

place it 90° to the bolster. You may find that the bolster is not tall enough for you, in which case add another long-fold blanket on top of the bolster to increase the height.

FIGURE 9.12

Sit on your knees next to the bolster facing out from the wall as shown in figure 9.13, with your right hip joint about in line with the middle of the bolster.

Lean forward and carefully roll over like you are rolling over in bed. Be sure you do not push yourself outward at all; just roll sideways. As you do so, swing your legs up the wall.

The key to the pose is that your tailbone should be at the far edge of the bolster, or better yet, slightly hanging over the edge of the bolster that is near the wall. You should be in an arch, which means that your lower front ribs are spreading apart.

Make sure that the C7 cervical vertebra is not pressing the floor but is slightly lifting up. Also be aware that your pelvis is positioned higher than

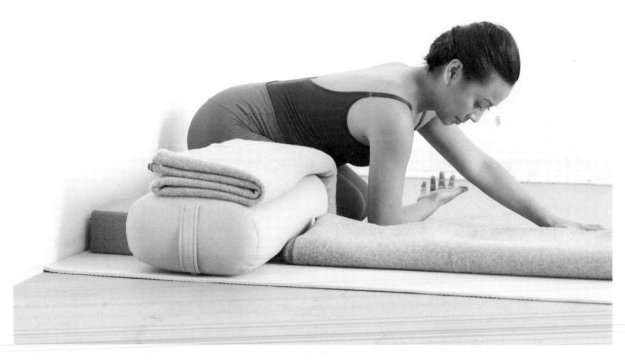

FIGURE 9.13

your heart, and your heart is above your head. Your trunk should not be flat but opened in a backbend as well as opening from side to side.

Once you are comfortable here, you need to do two things for the legs. First have a folded blanket ready. Now bend your knees and put a belt around your legs just beyond your kneecaps, that is, on the upper shinbone. Make the belt firm around the legs to help support them and hold them up easily in the pose. This will help you relax more.

The second thing to do before you straighten all the way is to put the folded blanket over your feet so that when you straighten the legs and place the heels on the wall, the heels will be comfortable. This blanket also keeps the feet warm. Now let your arms open naturally to the side.

Cover the rest of your body with an open blanket if you wish. Place the eye cover over your eyes. Remain in the pose for up to fifteen minutes. But do come down if you begin to feel pins and needles in your feet.

While you are in this powerful pose, let yourself be held by the props. Let go of all the thinking, planning, and doing, especially thinking about doing for others. The perimenopausal years are often very busy for most women who find themselves taking care of a family, perhaps raising teenagers, or letting go as children leave the nest, working part or full time, and even

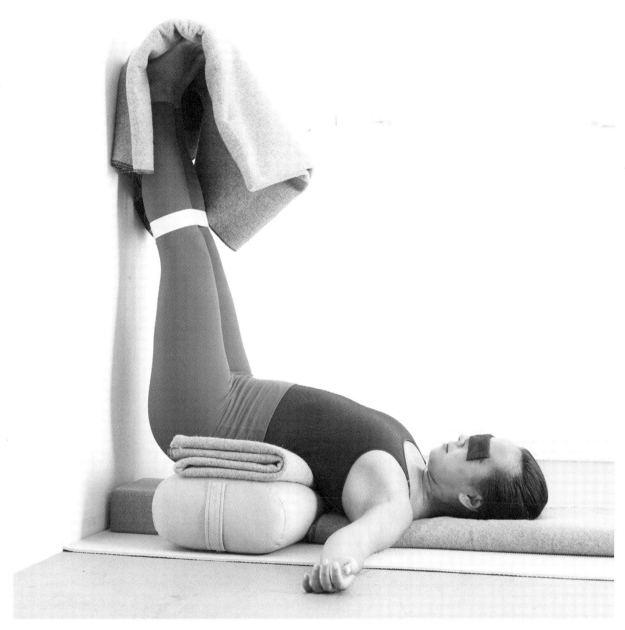

FIGURE 9.14

caring for aging parents. Think of VK as a mini vacation during which the pose becomes your refuge.

To come down, bend your knees, remove the blanket from the feet, and undo the belt. You can either roll to your side or gently push away from the wall until your pelvis is on the floor, then roll to the side and sit slowly up. Perhaps VK will give you a rest and a slightly new perspective on your day and your life.

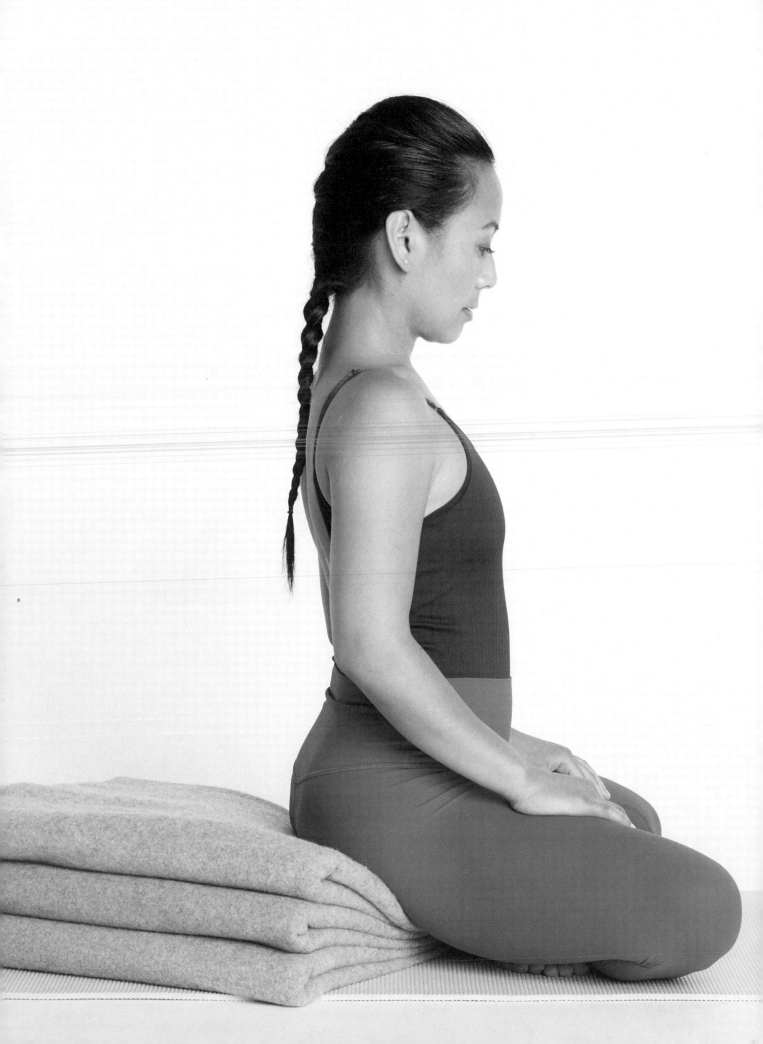

10

Dancing with the Breath

DIAPHRAGMATIC BREATHING AND OTHER MYTHS ABOUT BREATHING

The breath is the messenger between the body and the mind.

THE FIRST TIME I had the experience of how much power my breath had to affect my mind, I had not even heard of yoga. It was the winter of my third and last year of undergraduate school, and it was the final exam period in January. I had four finals in four days, somehow accidentally arranged exactly in descending order, beginning with my hardest exam and ending with my easiest.

When I walked into the classroom to take the last of the four exams, it was the final for my favorite class with my favorite professor. I knew the material cold. But when the professor passed out the exams and the blue books for us to write our answers in, something happened. When I read the exam questions, my mind went completely blank. That had never happened to me before, and it was probably a side effect of all the late hours and lack of sleep I had experienced in preparation for exams.

When I read the questions, nothing rang a bell. Literally I remembered nothing about the course that I had enjoyed so much for several months. But for some unknown reason, maybe because of a random blessing bestowed by a friendly Universe, I did not panic. I just folded my arms on my desk, learned forward and put my head down on my arms, and began to take long slow breaths.

My professor walked over and softly inquired as to my well-being. Assuring him I was okay, I stayed in that position, and just breathed with awareness for about ten minutes. Then I sat up, opened my blue book, and began to write.

All that I had learned and studied flowed out, and in the end, I maintained my high grade in the class.

But the real lesson, that my breath and mind were intimately connected and that I could "change" my mental state by breathing, was forgotten before I even turned in my blue book and left the building.

It was to be two more years before I reacquainted myself with the amazing power of the breath in my first yoga class. The awareness of breath, and breathing practices, were to become a daily part of my life as my yoga practice developed over the decades. I am still learning about this physical function that has the ability and profound power to change my mind and moods.

Why You Need to Know This

Breathing is a unique autonomic function. We can completely forget about it all day, and we certainly forget it when we sleep. Nonetheless, the process of breathing continues to provide oxygen to our cells and to release carbon dioxide on exhalation no matter what.

On the other hand, we can give our breath our full attention so we can hold it when we concentrate or go underwater, or use it to manipulate the mind as I did in the story above or to practice the yoga breathing technique called pranayama. What is so interesting to me about the breath is that it is a communication pathway between our mind and our body that we can trust to keep us alive and forget about most of the time. But it also is a communication pathway that we can deliberately manipulate at will. Both possibilities exist at the same time.

By contrast, we cannot do this with our heart. The heart beats from the earliest weeks of our life in our mother and for all the days that we live. We can learn to slow down the heart, but we really cannot control the heartbeat to the extent that we can our breath.

Pranayama, the yoga practice focused on the breath, is the fourth limb of the "eight limbed" yoga presented by Patanjali in his Yoga Sutras (Pada 2, verses 29 and 49–53). Pranayama, not surprisingly, is placed between the third limb, asana or physical posture, and the fifth limb, a state of mental awareness called *pratyahara*, meaning the conscious mental withdrawal from the input of the senses.

This placement is no doubt deliberate because the techniques of regulating the breath are very useful for changing states of mind by using a physical technique to create mental changes. But there is an additional component beyond just the physiological aspects of changing one's breath. Ancient yoga wisdom teaches that pranayama practice is also about energy.

One way to look at this is to unpack the Sanskrit word *pranayama* itself. *Prana* means, of course, "energy," and *yama* means "restraint." Thus, a more subtle definition of the word *pranayama* is that this practice is about conserving, directing, and using one's breath to channel prana for the desired physical, emotional, and mental effects. The desired effects are about creating a body-mind that is not only healthy but also a more finely tuned instrument for experiencing higher states of consciousness.

Patanjali teaches specifically in Pada 2, verse 51 of his Yoga Sutras, that with the practice of pranayama, the breath can potentially become almost still. The core of pranayama practice is paradoxically to slow and quiet the breath, not to increase it. With this slowing and quieting, the body and mind are profoundly affected.

Yet so many students of yoga seem to believe that the "goal" of pranayama is to breathe deeper and deeper and to actively hold the breath longer and longer, when the opposite is what is taught in the traditional teachings.

In fact, after many years of practice, I have experienced, as have many others, that when one practices pranayama, the breath at times seems to almost disappear, and one is left with a residue of profound stillness in both body and mind.

Whether one is a yoga student or teacher or neither, I believe it is important to understand the power you possess at any moment to use your breath to connect with yourself, to calm down, to help subdue a panic attack, to help you give birth, to meditate, to practice yoga asana, and sometimes to help lessen your experience of pain.

The breath is an eternal mantra, always rising and falling. One of the best meditations I know of is to simply watch this rising and falling. This practice of observing the breath can be done on the yoga mat or in the car. The location does not matter, because the breath is always there, available to be observed, available to be honored, and available to teach us about our inner state at this and every other moment. The breath therefore is always the potential teacher and provides us with the ever-present "yoga mat." The breath needs nothing more than your attention to be of value at any point during your day.

I believe that watching the breath is the highest form of pranayama practice because it does not involve any form of control. All desire and attempts to control it always come directly from our ego. Dispassionately watching the breath with absolutely no agenda is likely the most powerful thing we can do to bring ourselves into the radical present.

Breathing plays a part in all systems of Hatha yoga during the practice of asana. We are taught to inhale and exhale in coordination with our movements into and out of each asana. Sometimes we are instructed to hold the pose for a certain number of breaths. Breathing is the focus in the practice of pranayama and the same is often true during meditation. Most systems of meditation instruct their practitioners in some form of breath awareness and/or manipulation.

The breath is a manifestation of our first and most profound connection with life. You might even say breathing is life itself. During birth, life welcomes us with the gift of breathing. At the time of death, as our breathing slowly stops, it becomes the gentle wind that carries us through a portal into what I call the "trusted unknown." Practicing simple pranayama every day will change your mental state during the breathing practice itself, but it will also leave benevolent footprints on your mind and soul that will gradually change your life.

Your Structure

Breathing requires a wonderful ballet of coordination among your nervous system, blood chemistry, and muscular system. The respiratory system is made up of the nose, mouth, pharynx, larynx, trachea, bronchi, bronchioles, lungs, and alveoli, which are the small sacs in the lungs where gas exchange actually occurs.

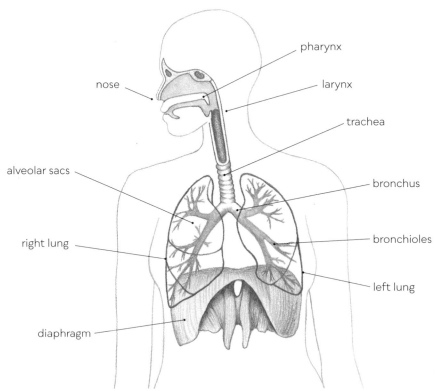

FIGURE 10.1

Notice how much of our lungs are in the side of the body and how much are in the back body. Actually, some estimates are that up to 60 percent of our lung tissue is in the back of our body. Remember that in the front of the chest cavity, the heart takes up a lot of space, and the lungs have to share that space with it.

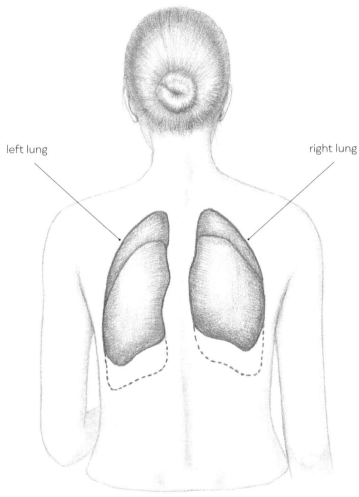

left lung

right lung

FIGURE 10.2
Posterior view of lungs

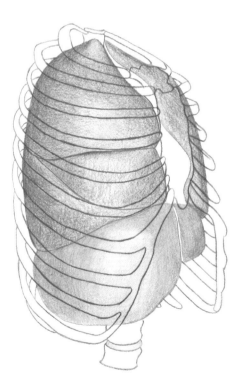

FIGURE 10.3
Lateral (side) lungs

The central muscle of respiration is the diaphragm. It divides the thorax, or chest, and the abdomen, into two distinct cavities. It is able, like the heart, to contract virtually nonstop twenty-four hours a day without fatiguing. It only rests very briefly after each exhalation.

The diaphragm is attached to the xiphoid process at the end of the sternum, to the costal cartilage of ribs 7–10, laterally to ribs 11 and 12, and the bodies of the first three lumbar vertebrae and the arcuate ligaments. It inserts onto itself at its most internal structure, called the central tendon, which ascends and fuses with the interior surface of the pericardium, the fascial sac of the heart.

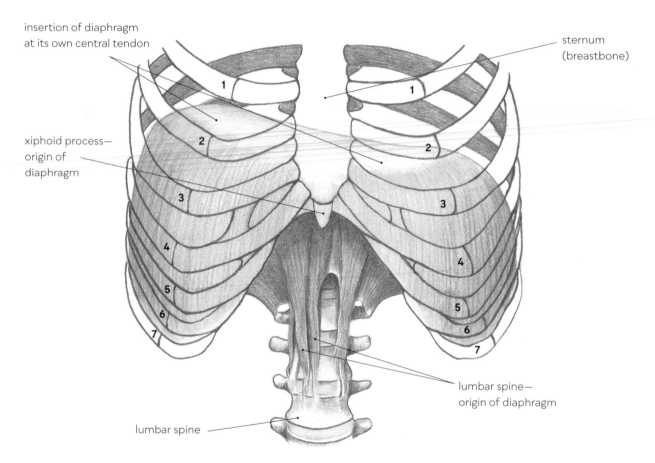

insertion of diaphragm at its own central tendon

sternum (breastbone)

xiphoid process— origin of diaphragm

lumbar spine— origin of diaphragm

lumbar spine

FIGURE 10.4
Diaphragm—origin and insertion

Knowing this, you can imagine how posture might affect your diaphragm. If the chest is dropped, and the vertebral column is in flexion, the excursion (movement up and down) of the diaphragm will be impeded. You can easily prove this to yourself by slumping, either in standing or sitting, and then try to take a deep easy breath. Your slumped posture directly impedes the ability of the diaphragm to move up and down.

Because of the diaphragm's connection to three lumbar vertebrae and to the rib cage, standing in Mountain Pose while tucking and distorting the curves of both the thoracic spine (source of the ribs) and the lumbar spine will directly interfere with breathing, just like slumping. This is just another reason not to tuck your tailbone in Mountain Pose or to sit with a flexed or rounded back, for that matter. (See chapter 1 for a review of the normal curves in Mountain Pose.)

The diaphragm, as stated above, is the primary muscle of respiration. Contraction of the diaphragm is the driving force that creates inhalation, during which the diaphragm descends. This muscular action of the diaphragm is created by the stimulation of the phrenic nerves. The word *phrenic* is related to the word *frantic*, which is how we can feel if we cannot take in sufficient air.

In normal quiet breathing, when we need to exhale, it is the natural recoil of the diaphragm after full inhalation that creates exhalation. However, in more active respiration, the relaxation of the secondary muscles of respiration, to the degree that they have been recruited, also help to create exhalation.

The secondary muscles of breathing include the abdominal muscles, the external and internal intercostal muscles, the serratus posterior superior and inferior, and the quadratus lumborum.

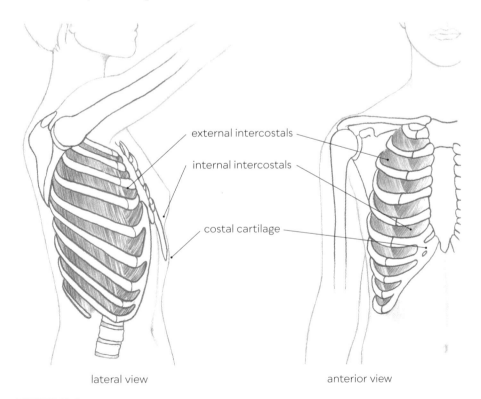

external intercostals

internal intercostals

costal cartilage

lateral view

anterior view

FIGURE 10.5
Intercostals

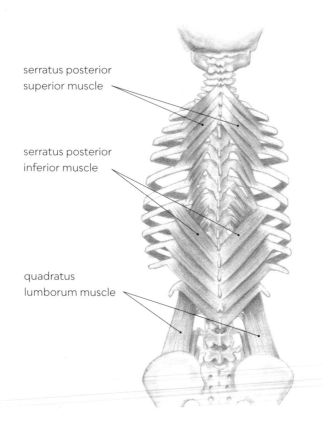

serratus posterior
superior muscle

serratus posterior
inferior muscle

quadratus
lumborum muscle

The quadratus and the serratus muscles help to pull the ribs down or up, depending on their specific location.

The abdominal muscles are active in forced exhalation, for example when we are running and need to exhale quickly. They are also engaged when we cough and aid in cases where there is lung disease, and the natural elasticity of the lungs is reduced. Other muscles like the pectoralis and the upper trapezius can also aid in respiration. But in quiet breathing, we almost exclusively use the diaphragm to exhale.

FIGURE 10.6
Posterior view of secondary respiratory muscles

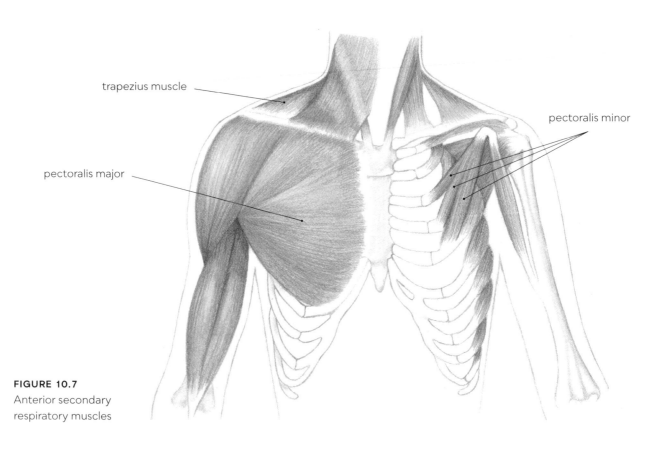

trapezius muscle

pectoralis minor

pectoralis major

FIGURE 10.7
Anterior secondary respiratory muscles

Your Anatomy in Action

Contraction of the diaphragm is the driving force that creates inhalation and is controlled by the phrenic nerves. The phrenic nerves are stimulated by the respiratory center in the brain stem where cells measure elevated levels of carbon dioxide in the bloodstream. When the respiratory center detects high carbon dioxide in the blood, the phrenic nerves stimulate the start of the respiratory cycle by causing the diaphragm muscle to contract. The carbon dioxide is then off-loaded from the blood to the lungs, and exhaled. Then the cycle starts all over again.

But we never exhale all the air out of the lungs. There is a residual volume of air maintained in the lungs while we are alive that is about one and a quarter quarts of volume. The volume of air that comes in and out during inhalation and exhalation is called the tidal volume, and it can change with exertion.

When the diaphragm is stimulated to contract by the phrenic nerves, the diaphragm muscle fibers contract so it shortens inward toward the central tendon. This causes the diaphragm actually to *descend*, pressing down on the abdominal organs and massaging them and the kidneys that are attached to the diaphragm. This descent creates more space in the thorax, which encourages the lungs to expand and air to rush into the lungs where the pressure has been reduced in relationship to pressure outside the body. When the oxygen in the lungs has been transferred into the bloodstream in the alveolar sacs of the lungs to be delivered to all the body's cells, the phrenic nerves stop firing.

Remember that it is the rising carbon dioxide level in the blood, not a low oxygen level, that drives the cycle of respiration. Taking a deep breath does encourage full oxygen exchange. However, it does not change gas diffusion within the lungs or affect blood oxygenation levels when the lungs are healthy and the air quality is good. The oxygen saturation level stays quite stable in your bloodstream, whether you are sleeping or running a marathon. If this level drops because of shallow breathing habits, high altitude, or compromised lung function caused by disease, you can become very ill.

It is a yoga myth that increasing inhalation puts more oxygen in your bloodstream. Again, for the student with healthy lungs and normal, relaxed breathing patterns, depth of breath does not increase oxygen in your bloodstream. What we can really manipulate is the level of carbon dioxide. My theory is that slowing the breath in pranayama practice helps us "learn" to tolerate slightly higher levels of carbon dioxide in our bloodstream, thus slowing down the respiratory cycle by retraining the brain not to be so quick to initiate respiration. This is just a theory, but it would be an interesting experiment to conduct. Whether it is an accurate theory or not, it is true that pranayama practice definitely slows down breathing rates gradually over time to six to ten breaths per minute in quiet breathing. And there is some evidence that this slowing is quite beneficial to health.[6]

In quiet breathing, the natural recoil of the diaphragm and the relaxation of the secondary muscles of respiration, to the degree that they have been recruited to aid inhalation, cause exhalation. Using the natural recoil of the diaphragm to create exhalation requires less metabolic energy expenditure since forced exhalation is not necessary in most daily activities.

When an increased rate of oxygen-carbon dioxide exchange is needed, like during running or dancing, for example, then the secondary muscles of respiration are recruited, mainly to aid in exhalation in a more rapid or more forced manner.

It is important to understand that the act of quiet breathing like we practice in pranayama does *not* really involve the pushing of the abdomen outward. There is a common yoga myth that when we push out the abdomen during breathing practice, we are doing "diaphragmatic breathing." My joke is to ask the rhetorical questions: Isn't all breathing diaphragmatic? Can you breathe without using your diaphragm?

I will agree that when we are lying down and breathing in a relaxed manner, there is a soft and slight movement of the abdomen up and down, but this is not what I am describing. I have seen yoga students aggressively push out their abdomen, so the bulge is quite large, during inhalation. Sometimes they actually look several months pregnant in the process. But anatomical reality teaches us that there are no lungs in the abdomen.

When I see this type of practice, I also tend to see that there is minimal movement in their rib cage during breathing. It is a simple anatomical fact that wherever there are ribs in the body, there are lungs. Stretching the intercostal muscles during the practice of asana can help breathing practice because intercostals, which are flexible, allow the rib cage to expand more easily with each inhalation and have perhaps a stronger natural recoil of the ribs on exhalation. But bulging out the abdomen does not expand the ribs at all and has great potential to actually weaken the abdominal wall.

Another objection I have to this technique of bulging out the abdomen in pranayama practice is that anatomically, about 60 percent of our lung tissue is in the back body. I like to instruct my students in gaining an awareness of and a facility with opening their side and back ribs in breathing practice to allow the lungs to expand to their maximum ability. This to me seems to be a much more effective way to breathe than pushing out the abdomen.

But yoga is an experiential practice first and foremost. My request is that you try the breathing practices offered below with awareness, ease, and an open mind. Learning to breath by focusing a little more on your rib cage instead of bulging out your abdomen hopefully will soon begin to feel more natural and more pleasant. I predict you will enjoy living in harmony with your body's wisdom around breathing.

MAIN POINTS TO REMEMBER FROM THIS CHAPTER

→ Breathing is a profound expression of our body-mind connection.

→ Breathing is an automatic function but can be overridden so the breath can be consciously manipulated.

→ Taking a deep breath does not increase the amount of oxygen in your bloodstream.

→ Carbon dioxide levels in the blood control the respiratory cycle.

→ Putting your attention on your breath at any time in your day will help improve your ability to be self-aware and reduce stress and thus calm you down.

→ There are no lungs in the abdomen.

Attentive Practice

It is easy to overlook the power that comes from a few minutes of conscious breathing. Besides the formal practices given below, one can take a few minutes while waiting in the car for someone or before turning on the computer in the morning to settle into watching the breath move.

One of my favorite times to do this informal practice is in my seat on the airplane, from the time when taxiing begins on the runway until we are airborne. Whenever you can, remember to watch your breath. This is especially interesting as a practice when you are feeling disgruntled and agitated. If you can watch your breath during these rough times, you will be amazed how quickly you move out of that stuck place.

CAUTIONS

The practices offered here are quite gentle. Of course, do not practice if you have a cold or a respiratory flu or worse. Remember that there is never to be a sense of strain when you practice; let go of the ambition of breathing deeper and deeper. Instead, learn to pay attention to increasing the fluidity with which you breathe and the smoothness you create as you move from inhalation to exhalation to inhalation.

If you want to go further with pranayama practice, find an experienced teacher. Even though the practices presented here are basic, be sure to check with your health-care provider before starting a practice if you have any of the following conditions:

- Asthma
- Uncontrolled high blood pressure
- COPD (chronic obstructive pulmonary disease)
- Any other significant lung disease

PROPS NEEDED

- Sturdy chair (optional)
- Nonslip yoga mat
- Five to six yoga blankets
- Bolster
- Eye cover
- Timer

The first two practices presented below fall under a category I call "breathing awareness" practices. They are designed to help you get in touch with the mechanics of breathing and to help you feel how your ribs actually move when you breathe. The final two practices are basic formal pranayama practices.

Some students enjoy practicing one or more of these breathing practices early in the morning before any other yoga. Others like to practice them at the end of an active asana practice to lead the body-mind naturally toward Deep Relaxation Pose. Still others prefer to separate their breathing practices entirely from the practice of yoga asana, for example, as a practice in the mid- or late afternoon. Whichever time you practice, make sure your stomach is not too full, and you are warm and comfortable in a quiet and inviting place.

Breathing Awareness
PRACTICE 1

This practice should be done sitting up at first. It can be done lying down as well using the same position that is offered for the Sama Vritti pranayama below after you feel comfortable with the sitting version.

Begin by sitting in a comfortable chair so that your vertebral column is in its natural curve. Remember that the diaphragm is connected to several lumbar vertebrae, therefore any slumping will interfere with the ability of the diaphragm to move. If you are in a chair, this usually means that you will be sitting close to the front edge of the chair, with your feet on the floor so your column can be free, long, and in the natural curves, not straight.

You can also practice this by sitting on your yoga mat. Place two or more folded yoga blankets on your mat and sit on the corners of the blankets in an easy cross-legged position. Observe the model in figure 10.8. Notice how she is *not* sitting on the edge, but exactly on the corners of the blankets so that her thighs can drop down. Note especially how her lower back is curved into her body, which is the normal curve for the lumbar spine. If the lumbar spine and pelvis are in neutral, they will set the stage for the rest of the spine, including the neck, to be comfortable.

Once you are comfortably settled, drop your chin slightly and close your eyes. Now place your hands, palms down, on the side of your lower ribs, a little above the last ribs. Your thumbs point backward, and your other fingers point forward.

Slowly begin to inhale through your nose and feel what is happening under your hands. You probably feel your side ribs are lifting and flaring outward. If you have your index fingers slightly

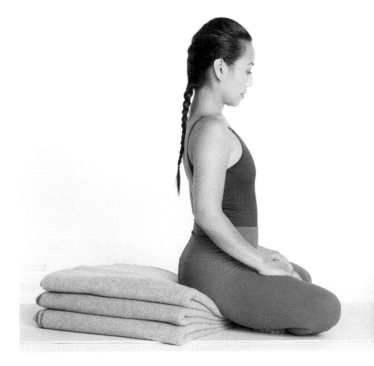

FIGURE 10.8

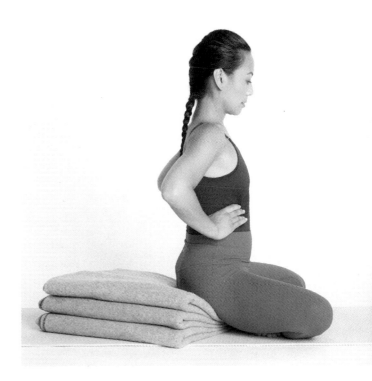

FIGURE 10.9

on the front of your rib cage and your thumbs more on the side of your rib cage, you will also feel that your rib cage is opening toward the front and back simultaneously.

Continue this for several breaths. Then try thinking of only breathing into your right lung. Without bending or shifting your vertebral column, you concentrate on breathing only into your right lung. After several breaths, switch to the left lung. Then breathe evenly with both lungs for several breaths, remembering to move all your ribs evenly before you stop. It is not necessary to try to maximize the amount you take in and give off; just breathe a little more than a normal breath so that you feel focused and comfortable.

Finally, release your hands and place them on your top thighs in a comfortable position with your palms facing *inward*. Now try a few simple long, slow breaths, focusing all your attention on breathing into your side body. You may want to place your hands back on your low side ribs and try again.

End with simply sitting, letting your breath remain simple and normal, with your hands on your thighs, and then reflect on your inner sense of calm. It is also lovely to follow these few moments of reflection with a twenty-minute Deep Relaxation Pose. For suggestions on how to practice Deep Relaxation Pose, see chapter 11.

Breathing Awareness
PRACTICE 2

This practice will bring awareness into your back body, where so much of the lungs are located. Begin by gathering your props: your yoga mat, a bolster—the longer the better—and a blanket for some padding under your head. You will also need another blanket to roll and place under your ankles.

Place your bolster on your mat and lie face down on your belly. Place your arms out to your sides in a way that is comfortable for you and rest your feet on a thick rolled-up towel or small bolster, whichever feels more comfortable on your lower back. Most students like to hang the head downward, but use a blanket as a bit of a pillow if you want. This position should be quite comfortable.

Begin, as we always do with any form of breathing practice, by just watching your breath. Then begin to actively invite the breath to move into your back body as much as possible on each inhalation. You might be surprised at how much breathing is happening in the back of the rib cage.

Take long, slow, easy breaths. Remember that it is important that you never push yourself when practicing. You do not want to feel agitated, restless, or winded. Slowly and steadily, with your mind, direct your breath to the back of your body. Remember that 60 percent of the lungs are here. Notice that not only is your back body moving with your breath, but your back side waist is moving as well.

After a few breaths, stop and just be still. Notice your mind. Then try again for several breaths. When you are done, carefully roll or slide off your bolster and lie on your back on the floor. Take five slow breaths while keeping your awareness on breathing into your back body. Practice Deep Relaxation Pose for twenty minutes.

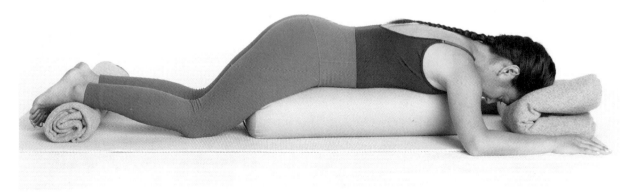

FIGURE 10.10

Sama Vritti

PRANAYAMA PRACTICE 1

The word *sama* means "equal" and the word *vritti* means "disturbance." This is another way of saying "harmony," because harmony is a disturbance we like. Thus, this pranayama is about making all four parts of the breath—inhalation, retention, exhalation, and retention—the same. However, in the practice presented here, we will only focus on even inhalation and even exhalation.

You may not realize it, but when we are not conscious of our breathing during a normal day, the breath is not really even. I learned this when I was fulfilling one of my internships in order to complete my training to become a physical therapist.

When I worked with an experienced respiratory therapist as part of my training to become a physical therapist, she told me that breathing machines were set to have an uneven breath every now and again. This was done so that the machines would more accurately replicate normal human breathing when they were being used to help patients.

So, the idea of making the breaths exactly even for an extended period is a form of "yama" or restraint. That is one reason I call this a pranayama practice and not a breathing practice. In breathing practices, we are more about observing the natural breath then attempting to control it in a particular way.

Begin by setting up the props as shown in figure 10.11.

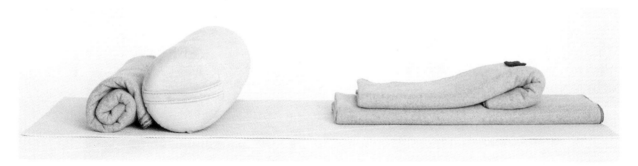

FIGURE 10.11

The idea is to elevate the head slightly higher than the chest, and the chest slightly higher than the abdomen. Place the bolster under your knees so that it supports the back of your knees specifically and does not lift the thighs. The tops of your thighs at the hip joint should be clearly dropping down. The rolled blanket under the ankles should lift the heels slightly from the floor. The feet should float. Again, be specific with your propping. The ankle support is only for the Achilles tendon. Please make sure your knees are twice as high as your ankles.

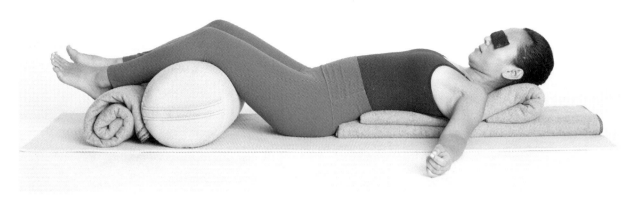

FIGURE 10.12

Sit very close to the end of your two long-fold blankets. There should be no gap between your body and the two blankets. Your body should be snugly pressed against your blankets. But neither should you sit on the blankets. Instead, sit on your mat. The blankets are to support the lumbosacral spine.

Lie back and reach up and turn the end of the top blanket under to support your head and neck. The support of your neck should actually extend under your trunk a bit and not stop midneck. Make sure your chin is slightly lower than your forehead. Cover up with a blanket, put on your eye cover, and then slide your arms under the blanket and position them wide open to the side. Your armpits should be open so that your inner upper arm does not touch the side of your ribs, even a little bit.

The first thing to do when you lie down is to spend the first minute or two making sure that you are totally comfortable, then spend at least five to ten minutes relaxing. It is very important that you are relaxed when you practice pranayama. An ancient teaching says that when you practice pranayama, the more still and silent you are on the inside, the more powerful the practice will be for your nervous system.

When you are completely relaxed, start to watch your breath. As much as possible, do not change it in any way. Do not try to make it longer or more even. Just observe it with neutrality. This may take a while to perfect.

To begin the practice, slowly inhale; you may want to make a slight sound from the back of your throat as you do this. This sound is created by imagining that you are breathing from the base of your throat, that the "nose is in the throat." The noise you hear should be just loud enough for you, and you alone, to hear.

This is the noise of a type of pranayama called *ujjayi* breath and can be a very effective point of focus. Remember, the sound should be very subtle and grow even more subtle as you continue in the pranayama practice. No one near you should be able to hear it at all. This is not about creating a rough sounding breath but rather one that is as smooth as the finest silk.

Imagine that this first breath is filling about half of your lungs. At the height of inhalation, there should be a natural pause before you begin to slowly exhale. Let the translation of inhalation into exhalation be slow, soft, and steady, with no jerks. Likewise, at the end of exhalation there is a slight pause as well. Do not "clamp" down or hold in in any way with the abdomen; just be fully present with the very brief pause before you begin your next inhalation.

Now take a normal breath in, a normal breath out. Then begin to draw in another long, slow pranayama breath, this time taking in slightly more air than before and letting out the exact same amount but with no jerks or bumps in the process of the breath. It should take at least three or four long pranayama inhales and exhales before you feel as if you are able to fill your lungs to about 75 percent of your maximum. The lung tissue needs to be gently stretched with the breath, just like the intercostal muscles between your ribs need to be gently stretched. Take your time and proceed with gentleness.

Remember the practices given above about breathing from the ribs? Do that now. During the inhalation, imagine that you are lifting your side ribs up and then out and inviting your lungs to follow. This will issue an invitation to the breath to come and find your lungs. The ribs are the creator of inhalation, and the lungs follow.

To exhale, imagine your lungs are separating away from the inner lining of the rib cage and are gently squeezing your breath out while the ribs float down to a resting position. The key is to remember that with each breath, your inhalation is created by the ribs, your exhalation is created by the lungs. At least this is how I recommend you think about it. Actually this all happens at once, but thinking about it this way will not only give you a focal point but will draw the mind down into the chest and away from the external world.

Take another normal breath in, followed by a normal breath out. Do one or two of these shorter normal breaths between *every* long inhale and exhale. There is no need to try to make the pranayama breaths as long as you can.

Be tender with yourself. The most important thing is *not* the quantity of breath, but the quality. Continue to spread the ribs on inhale and squeeze the lungs on exhale. When you practice this way, there will be minimal movement in the abdomen.

When using your side ribs in this manner feels comfortable, begin to add the back body to your focus as well. Now not only will you lift your side ribs on inhalation, you will also breathe into the back body. Remember most of the lung tissue is there.

Practice this pranayama following this particular order: watch the breath, deepen and slow the inhalation by opening the side ribs and the back lungs.

Exhale by moving your lungs toward the center of your thorax, like a round balloon letting out air moves toward its center. After this long breath, take a normal shorter inhale and exhale to refresh you. Remember not to bulge out your abdomen during this pranayama; there are no lungs in the abdomen! Breathe wherever there are ribs, because where there are ribs, there are lungs.

At no point is there any sense of ambition, strain, or effort. Your mind has deeply retreated to the center of your head, your body is totally relaxed, and your breath is a natural rising and falling that captures all your attention.

If at any time during this practice you feel breathless or agitated, release the breath to its own intelligence for a while and then begin again. Often the way you know you need to stop and begin again is when it seems harder and harder to keep the exhalation exactly the same from the beginning of exhalation to the end of exhalation.

If there are any jerks, or there is any sense of "breath hunger," breathe quietly for a while. When you begin again, make the inhalation shorter and match it exactly with an exhalation. If you think about it, it makes sense to consider a slowed-down exhalation as a form of retention. Slowing down the exhalation actually causes us to retain more carbon dioxide in the lungs, and if we are unable to keep the exhalation completely easy at the very end, we are doing too much for us at that moment. Please practice by listening to your body and progressing slowly with your pranayama practice.

After about ten to fifteen minutes of practice (you may want to set an alarm), let the breath completely alone and once again simply watch it. If you are still comfortable in this position, stay and practice a twenty-minute Deep Relaxation Pose.

Or if you prefer, practice one of the variations of Deep Relaxation Pose presented in chapter 11. Whether you stay as you are or choose another Deep Relaxation Pose variation, as you begin a formal relaxation practice, take a few minutes to just reflect on how your breath may have changed, on how your body feels, and on the state of your mind. When Deep Relaxation Pose is over, inhale, and roll to your side of choice as you exhale. Lie there for a few minutes and use your arms to help you slowly sit up.

I recommend practicing this Sama Vritti breath for at least six months before trying the Visama Vritti practice below. I consider Sama Vritti the "Mountain Pose" of pranayama practice. If you have been away from your practice, have been traveling or ill, or have been under great stress, come back home to Sama Vritti. Only add Visama Vritti when the conditions are more spacious in your life.

Pranayama practice is much more subtle than asana practice, and the progress in pranayama, unlike the progress in asana, cannot be so easily seen. I like to say that progress in asana practice is a steep curve of improve-ment in the beginning, but over the years that curve begins to flatten out. Pranayama practice is exactly the opposite. In the beginning when one takes on a regular pranayama practice, the improvement is subtle and seems very slow, almost undetectable. But if you are faithful to your practice, the curve of improvement, while starting as a very slow rise (almost a flat line), will begin to move up steeply, and that improvement will become just as obvious as the improvement in asana practice.

Your friends can see your asana progress, but you can feel your pranayama progress in the stability of your mental state and in your lack of reactivity to life's irritations. This will become more and more apparent to you as you practice pranayama regularly over time.

Visama Vritti
PRANAYAMA PRACTICE 2

This practice is similar to the previous one in some ways but varies in that the exhalation is longer than the inhalation: *visama* means "uneven." After you have practiced Sama Vritti consistently for six months, try this next step.

Set yourself up in the exact position explained for Sama Vritti. When you are relaxed and settled, begin as you did previously. Start by watching your natural breath. Notice how this begins to calm you.

Once you feel at ease, proceed to create long, smooth inhalations followed by long, smooth exhalations. Take a normal breath in between each long inhale and exhale. Keep this rhythm for several minutes, gradually stretching the lungs with your breath, and focus on smooth transitions between the inhalations and the exhalations.

When you are ready, gradually extend your exhalation. For example, you might want to count slowly to four on your inhalation, and slowly to six on your exhalation. Then take at least one normal and less deep inhalation and exhalation. Then with the next breath, go back to a four to six ratio. You can gradually increase the timing of the inhalation and the exhalation, but you are always attempting to make the exhalation slightly longer.

Remember to use the ribs, especially the back and side ribs, to initiate inhalation, and to imagine that the lungs "contract" to initiate exhalation, so it feels that the ribs press down onto the lungs as you exhale. Thus, the exhalation feels more active than the inhalation. This is a visualization that many students find useful. Actually, all these processes are naturally occurring as they should and in their own intelligent rhythm.

Wherever there are ribs, there are lungs. Let go of the yoga myth that you need to breathe deeply into the abdomen. Keep your abdomen passive, though it will move naturally and slightly without your interference.

When you have spent about ten to fifteen minutes practicing Visama Vritti, let the breath begin to settle on its own and lie quietly. End your practice by watching the breath again. Then let go of any attempt to control your breath.

Either practice Deep Relaxation Pose where you are, in this propped-up position, or pick another version of Deep Relaxation Pose from chapter 11. Finally, after you have rested for twenty minutes, and as it feels appropriate, roll to your side of choice and use your arms to help you sit up slowly.

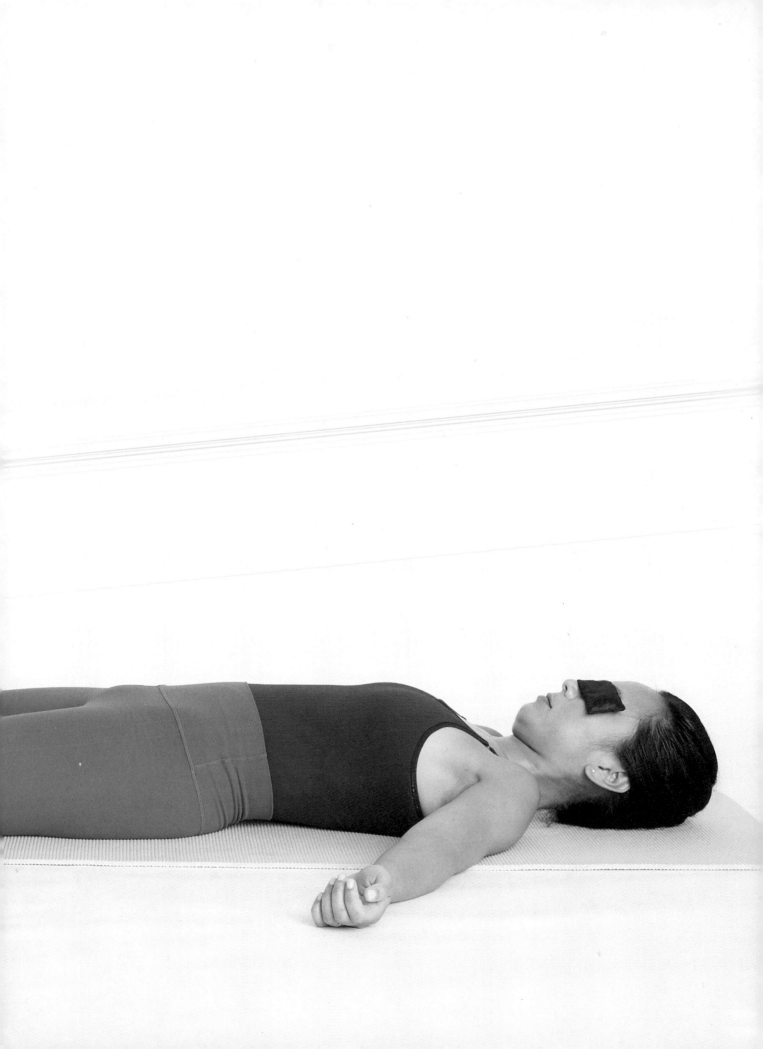

11

Deep Relaxation Pose (Savasana)

WHY DOING NOTHING FOR TWENTY MINUTES IS *NEVER* A WASTE OF TIME

To be still, silent, and receptive is to be at one with the Universe.

DEEP RELAXATION POSE (Savasana), also known as Corpse Pose, is not a pose that some people expect to end their yoga class with these days, as some styles of yoga asana do not teach it at all. I certainly did not expect it many years ago either, when I took my first yoga class. I thought lying down and resting was a waste of time when we could be up and doing more poses, stretching into more interesting shapes, and stroking the ego with impressive suppleness or strength.

This youthful period of my life had but one real problem: I had difficulty falling asleep almost every night. So when I finally was introduced to Deep Relaxation Pose, I was quite surprised that one could actually *choose* to relax on purpose. I thought that relaxing to prepare for sleep, if I thought about it at all, was something that just happened to you if you were lucky. Falling asleep was a mysterious thing that was beyond my ability to influence. But when I learned the skill of how to practice a purposeful, choice-full deep relaxation, I was hooked because my insomnia vanished, and my life got better.

Years later, I was teaching a workshop for teachers, and the class was about to end with Deep Relaxation Pose. Just for fun, I asked the teachers to raise their hands and tell me how long they kept their students in Deep Relaxation Pose at the end of their own weekly classes. The answers ranged from "Never;

I tell them to do it at home so we don't waste class time with it," to "Five or ten minutes, or maybe twelve minutes." Not one teacher in the class answered, "Twenty minutes," the time I actually recommend for the pose.

Then I asked everyone to close their eyes and to raise their hand if they regularly practiced Deep Relaxation Pose for at least fifteen to twenty minutes in their own practice. Almost no hands were raised. Remember, this was a class solely for yoga teachers. I was both saddened and surprised by this response, and the next day we discussed this outcome in our class when I shared with them the important reasons for a twenty-minute Deep Relaxation Pose. Perhaps this incident helped to feed my deep interest in the power of this pose, and in Restorative yoga in general.

Please do not get caught up in the yoga myth that Deep Relaxation Pose can be well practiced in five minutes or that it is not that important a pose to practice at all. In fact, I would go so far as to say that if you only have twenty minutes to practice yoga asana in a day, then choose Deep Relaxation Pose. The effects are so profound and so beneficial that I call this pose the "twenty-minute miracle." It will improve your health, reduce your stress, stimulate your creativity, and when practiced regularly, change your life.

Why You Need to Know This

Deep Relaxation Pose is never a waste of time. Never. Deep Relaxation Pose can revive your energy, lift your mood, give you a new perspective for the rest of your day, and reduce your stress.

One does not have to study the pervasive effects of stress for very long to discover that stress is considered a part of all illnesses and diseases. Stress is a major contributing factor to aging. Stress can make symptoms of any disease worse, it can increase the perception of pain, and it can actually change the telomeres, the protective covering at the end of each strand of DNA.

Stacy Lu states in the *American Psychological Association* article "How Chronic Stress Is Harming Our DNA":

> Each time a cell divides, it loses a bit of its telomeres. An enzyme called telomerase can replenish it, but chronic stress and cortisol exposure can decrease your supply of telomerase. When the telomere is too diminished, it often dies or becomes pro-inflammatory. This sets the aging process in motion, along with associated health risks.[7]

One of the best methods of slowing down aging and reducing anxiety and stress is by regularly practicing relaxation techniques such as Deep

Relaxation Pose. Unlike all drugs, legal and illegal, Deep Relaxation Pose does not have any deleterious side effects. All the side effects of the pose are beneficial for both body and mind.

Since 2001 I have been training yoga teachers in specific workshops how to teach Restorative yoga. I define Restorative yoga as "the use of props to support the body in positions of comfort and ease to facilitate relaxation and health." Those teachers who want to become certified in my approach to Restorative yoga must submit a project that involves setting up three of their students in restorative poses. They send me photos of those setups and an explanation of why they chose the poses, as well as a brief health history of each student.

For me, the best part of the project reports is reading the comments submitted by the students who have been set up by my trainees. I have read literally thousands of these comments, and they range from the fairly simple to the dramatic.

Here are a few examples: "After our session, I slept through the night for the first time in six months." "After our session my headaches went away." "After our session, and after practicing at home for a while, I had a normal menstrual period for the first time in years." "During the work week following our class together, I did not react to a difficult coworker; I stayed calm. This is huge for me." "Because of my Restorative practice, I have no more constipation." "After practicing Restorative yoga in the weeks since our session, my irritable bowel syndrome has gradually decreased and now appears to be gone." "Because of what I have learned and practiced with Restorative yoga, my chronic anxiety is greatly diminished and I may be able to go off medication." "Restorative yoga has helped me recover from extreme athletic competitions almost immediately with no soreness or tightness."

While these comments may seem surprising, they are not made up. What these people are reflecting in a very personal and individual way is that stress has consequences. Perhaps many of the "symptoms of modern life" that we accept as "normal" are really just the different ways each of us reacts to stress. Some of us react with anxiety, some of us with headaches, some of us with digestive disturbances, and others with a wide variety of other forms of dysfunction, discomfort, and pain.

In 2006 I was an advisor for a study conducted under the auspices of the National Institutes of Health to study the effect of Restorative yoga, including Deep Relaxation Pose, on hot flashes experienced by perimenopausal women. These women practiced forty-five minutes of Restorative yoga three times a week, two times in a class setting with a teacher, and once at home on their own.

At the end of the study, the women reported a reduction in the severity and frequency of their hot flashes. But blood tests confirmed other benefits. Some participants found the relaxation had reduced or stabilized their blood sugar levels. Others experienced a reduction in LDL cholesterol and triglyceride levels.

What seemed to be happening was that the regular practice of relaxation helped the participants to find a more balanced state of health. By decreasing their stress response, these women's bodies were able to find a physical state of homeostasis, or balance. In other words, when stress is reduced, the body is much more able to find its natural state, which is health.

There are many different Restorative poses, just like there are many different active asana. But I call Deep Relaxation Pose the "Mountain Pose" of Restorative yoga. Mountain Pose is the basic pose that is often taught at the beginning of yoga asana classes, and it's centered on the vertical line of our body and its relationship to gravity. Deep Relaxation Pose is the basic position of relaxation that has been taught since yoga asana has been practiced.

One of the many reasons I think that it is important to practice Deep Relaxation Pose at the end of an active asana class is that it gives the body time to integrate the active practice. It is almost like the body is "digesting" the effects of the active asana and weaving that new knowledge into the nervous system.

Deep Relaxation Pose is more than a closing ritual for a yoga class though. It is the bringing together of all the movements that have come before and creating out of them a new state of consciousness. Don't miss this delicious state of being.

Your Structure

You were probably your most relaxed when you were still in the womb. Perhaps part of the reason for this is that in the womb, all your joints are in flexion, that is, slightly bent. Maybe this is why we usually curl up all through our life when we are dozing off to sleep. Perhaps the brain, peripheral nervous system, muscles, and joints all "remember" the position of being in flexion from before birth and associate this position with safety. Whatever the reason, most people seem to enjoy Deep Relaxation Pose more when all their joints are propped into slight flexion. (See the "Attentive Practice" section below for instructions for practicing Deep Relaxation Pose with props.)

You may not realize that your joints have nerves that tell the central nervous system where your body is in space. These nerves are called proprioceptors, or position sense nerves. These nerves let us know where we are in space, and that helps us to adapt to gravity. It is my theory that propping your joints into flexion in Deep Relaxation Pose will stimulate the position sense nerves to tell your brain that it is safe to relax, just like in the womb.

Another way to use your structure to help you relax is to pay extra attention in Deep Relaxation Pose to the exact position of your head. Try this experiment. Sit with both feet on the floor, your pelvis evenly balanced on the more forward part of the chair, and your pubic bone slightly moving downward toward the chair. These three things should bring you in a position in which your spinal curves are in the perfect curves, or what anatomists call "normal curves" for the spinal column.

Make sure your eyes are looking straight ahead, not up or down, and that your head is balanced directly over your body. Also make sure you are not sitting with your head in a forward head posture. In other words, your head is now sitting exactly over your shoulders and is not jutting forward.

Now lift your chin slightly. Notice how your eyes tend to look upward and your attention goes up and away from your body. Now tilt the head slightly down. This time notice how your eyes follow your head, and your attention is naturally brought downward to a quiet, inward place.

The position of the head is critical when you are practicing Deep Relaxation Pose. Some students find that when they lie on the floor with no props, their head tends to hang or tilt backward quite a bit, and the chin is higher than the forehead. This could be related to the width of their rib cage from front to back. When the rib cage is thick from front to back, the head will hang backward by necessity. Other students find their head hangs backward because they have tight tissues in the back lower skull area and in the back of the neck. This happens when one sits and stands with forward head posture for years or even decades.

Whether or not your head tilts backward in Deep Relaxation Pose, it is always advisable to use some propping, usually a folded blanket, to lift the head so the chin can be slightly dropped. There is an important distinction to understand here.

The head and the neck are different structures. Of course they are connected. But many students seem more concerned with supporting the neck instead of the head. What these students tend to do is to put a rolled blanket or cloth under their neck, and they do not support their head. This strategy actually increases the cervical curve, and the head drops backward, and the chin lifts. This position, as you found above, tends to stimulate your brain, not quiet it.

The reason that is given for this propping strategy is to "protect the curve in the neck." But this reasoning does not take into account the fact that we are swimming in a sea of gravity, and our muscles, joints, and bones are always responding to that gravitational force. When one is standing or sitting up, the normal curve of the cervical spine is designed to hold the weight of the head, adapting all our movements to the downward force of gravity while we are in a vertical line.

But when you are lying down, as you are in Deep Relaxation Pose, the effect of gravity has been greatly decreased on the spinal structures of the neck, and the cervical spine flattens out a bit naturally. It is better to have your natural cervical curve maintained while standing. But once you are lying down this is not so true.

This is because there is minimal weight through the cervical spine in the horizontal position. So, flattening it a bit to drop the chin and induce introspection and relaxation is not a problem for the overwhelming number of students. It is highly likely that you really do not need to "support the curve in your neck" with a roll in Deep Relaxation Pose unless you have specific instructions from your health-care provider to do so.

If you can lie down now on your back, do so. Reach up and feel the back of your neck. Likely it will feel soft and relaxed. If you were to feel the back of your neck in standing, and created even the slightest forward head posture, you would notice a surprising amount of tension in the muscles of your posterior neck.

So when we are lying down, it is healthy to slightly tilt the chin down. This especially involves the upper cervical joints, i.e., the skull and C1 joint, and the C1 and C2 joint.

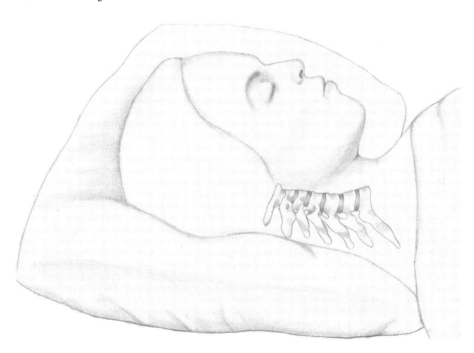

FIGURE 11.1
Cervical spine in slight flexion in Deep Relaxation Pose with head support

The rest of the neck in a propped Deep Relaxation Pose is slightly flattened, but no matter, because the neck is not holding up the head against the force of gravity; the head is being completely supported by the floor. This support allows us to lie in slight flexion with no strain to the neck.

Putting a roll under the middle of the back of the neck to "protect" the neck when lying down is a yoga myth. Placing a roll under the neck in Deep Relaxation Pose does not really do what some think it does. It actually arches or extends the neck, which means the chin comes up, and this tends to agitate the brain. When the chin is slightly dropped down in the pose, i.e., the cervical spine is in slight flexion, then the back of the neck is soft, the attention is drawn inward, and the brain is quieter. Remember, this is just slight flexion, and most of it comes from the upper cervical joints. We create this in Deep Relaxation Pose by paying attention to the position of our head first, then supporting the sides of the neck. More on how to do this later in this chapter.

So, the art of propping the body in Deep Relaxation Pose is really about manipulating the nervous system to relax deeply. If the word *manipulating* seems unpleasant to you, consider this. We are always manipulating our nervous system all day every day in so many ways. A few examples that we do this are that we take a shower, go for a run, drink coffee, stand on our head. And there are of course many other ways to manipulate our nervous system.

The salient question is: What kind of manipulation are we choosing, conscious or unconscious? Yoga is an ancient system that was created to manipulate the nervous system through practices like yoga asana, pranayama, and meditation in order to facilitate a radical change in perspective or consciousness so that we ultimately reduce our suffering and live in and understand the Truth of existence.

My fervent hope is that you choose, each and every day, to manipulate your nervous system into a state of deep relaxation. The residue in your body and mind from doing this will beneficially affect not only your life but also the lives of all those you come into contact with and, I believe, the whole planet.

Your Anatomy in Action

I define Deep Relaxation Pose as a pose in which the head and the heart are on the same level, or very close to it. In any type of asana practice, one might divide poses into two other categories: head above the heart and head below the heart. But in Deep Relaxation Pose we balance the brain and the heart, so it could be said that it is a more "neutral" asana.

The position of the head and the heart in relationship to gravity has effects on your organs. When you're sitting up, the brain begins to become measurably quieter when you recline backward to an angle of about 45° degrees. This is the familiar angle of a deck chair, lounge chair, or recliner. We know this angle intuitively when we sit in one of these reclining chairs, and we put it back to a comfortable recline. We also miss this angle when we are seated in an airplane seat that does not recline.

This physical reclining angle changes the brain by activating a nerve tract called the reticular activating system (RAS). The RAS is in charge of waking up other nerve tracts, and when we recline to 45° or more, the RAS begins to be less and less active. Thus we begin to experience the sense of relaxation when we begin to recline. This effect of the RAS with reclining posture is even stronger when we lie down to practice Deep Relaxation Pose and to sleep.

A yoga myth surrounding the practice of Deep Relaxation Pose is that the rest one gains from the pose is not needed if one sleeps adequately at night. However, the physiological truth is that rest and sleep are two distinct neurological states that can be clearly differentiated in brain studies. It turns out that to be truly healthy, we need both states. And in fact, students often find that when they take the time to rest in the daytime, they actually sleep better that night.

I often tell my classes to remember these four main factors when teaching or practicing Deep Relaxation Pose: still, quiet, dark, and warm. This is what our physiology needs to relax. We can improve the chances that students will relax in class when these four main factors are present.

To relax we must be still. The simple fact is that physical movement is stimulating to the nervous system. And it is hard to be still if we are not comfortable. That is why yoga props are so important when practicing. The props make us more comfortable.

The most important part of the body to prop is the head. If your head and neck are not comfortable, then you will not be able to go as deeply into the relaxation. In the "Attentive Practice" section below, there are instructions on how to prop your head and the rest of your body so that you are very comfortable; all your joints are in slight flexion, so that being still is all you want to do.

The second thing we need to encourage for the practice of Deep Relaxation Pose, is that we need quiet around us if we are to be able to let go deeply. This is why I do not talk when I am teaching Deep Relaxation Pose. I usually talk for two or three minutes at the very beginning of the pose, perhaps giving a simple breathing practice and/or some suggested instructions about letting the body go and the mind settle, but then I am quiet for the rest of the twenty minutes.

I do not believe that there is such a thing as a guided relaxation. If I am talking to you while you are lying in Deep Relaxation Pose, and if you are listening to me, then you are thinking my thoughts and integrating my images into your practice of Deep Relaxation Pose and not having your own experience of the pose. You are in effect being drawn outward and away from yourself toward my words and not moving inward toward your own center. Or you are tuning my words out, not listening at all, *so that you can have your own experience* of the pose. So why am I talking at all? My talking the whole time in Deep Relaxation Pose is not helping you deeply understand and experience the state of relaxation. I think the practice of leading or teaching during the practice of this pose is a yoga myth reflecting a major misunderstanding about how our physiology works. We simply need silence to relax.

I actually think that talking in Deep Relaxation Pose is more about the teacher's fear that she is not giving enough to her class, or that the students will become bored or agitated with silence. Actually silence is what we all need. It is in the silence that we can truly notice the agitations we call "mind." It is in this state of noticing that one begins to learn the most important thing a human being can learn: the difference between thoughts and consciousness. In the silent space of Deep Relaxation Pose, one can experience one's own consciousness, one's True Self, and settle there.

One can watch one's thoughts rise and fall, dance and twirl and agitate, but not go with them. This is a deep and powerful learning about who we really are and how we can be in the world. I call this state dis-identification. When we identify with our thoughts, we suffer. When we identify with our True Self, in that moment we are living in the eternal present and there is no suffering. Deep Relaxation Pose is often the first time many people have experienced this disidentification.

Darkness is the next factor to create. Light is one of the strongest stimuli to the brain. Have you ever been awakened by the full moon shining in your bedroom window? We are physiologically programmed to wake up with light and to rest with dark. This pattern is written in our very neurology from time out of mind.

Therefore, I strongly recommend that you use some form of covering for your eyes during Deep Relaxation Pose. Make sure that the covering does not press directly on the eyeballs themselves. Some yoga eye bags are so heavy that they can slightly indent the cornea, and when you come out of Deep Relaxation Pose, these slight impressions on your cornea might make it difficult for you to focus. This has happened to me and to many other yoga students. It may take a few minutes for your cornea to rehydrate and your vision to return to normal, but it is best not to create this occurrence in the first place.

Finally, we cannot relax if we are cold. When the periphery of the body, like the hands and feet are cold, the body does not know that you are not freezing to death. So the nervous system is roused to keep you awake. So, it is important to cover up in Deep Relaxation Pose.

I cannot tell you how many times I have heard students declare, "I don't need a blanket. I never get cold in Deep Relaxation Pose." These are the very students who reach over to get a blanket to cover themselves during the pose, usually about one minute before I ring my bells to announce the end of Deep Relaxation Pose.

I suggest you wear socks, if you wish, and cover your body, including your arms and your trunk. You will realize that staying for twenty minutes or more in the pose does produce a cooling down that actually can be counterproductive to relaxation.

There are other factors, of course, that facilitate relaxation, like a sense of safety, for example. For this reason, I let my students know that neither I, nor my assistants, will touch them during Deep Relaxation Pose. I do say that in the first five minutes one of us might whisper to them, asking permission to slightly adjust the head or their arms for example. But after that no one will disturb them.

I also let my new students know what the social context of this pose is. I remember clearly my first Deep Relaxation Pose. I kept lifting up my head and looking all around to see what was going on in all the silence. Tell your students that you all are practicing relaxation in a period of silence and explain to them how you will bring them out of the pose. I gently ring my bells to end the pose, but there are other techniques as well.

Paying attention to the effects that adequate propping and the "still, quiet, dark, and warm" mantra creates when you practice or teach Deep Relaxation Pose will enhance relaxation. Remember, we are manipulating the nervous system to create a different state of consciousness. This is a powerful technique. Practice it with intention, regularity, and respect for its power.

Attentive Practice

If I had to pick just one yoga asana to teach the world, it would be Deep Relaxation Pose. Anyone can practice it, though not everyone can get down on the floor or lie comfortably on the back. (Pregnant women should practice Side-Lying Deep Relaxation Pose, preferably on the left side as many doctors suggest. Please see the "Cautions" section below.)

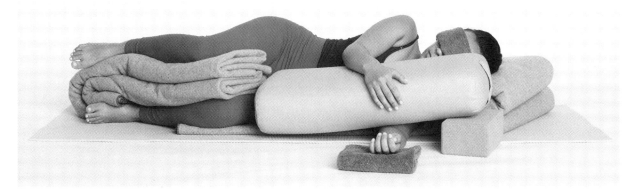

FIGURE 11.2

I have taught Deep Relaxation Pose in every kind of situation imaginable and have always found it to help the students, even if the props are not perfect or the room totally quiet.

Be creative in your use of props if there seem to be none available. I have used couch cushions and backpacks to prop legs, towels to prop heads, socks and washcloths to cover eyes, and coats to cover students. The important thing to do is to practice.

CAUTIONS

For those who cannot lie comfortably on their back, try to make the hard surface of the floor more comfortable. You can also elevate the legs to change where the weight is felt on your lower back.

Beginning the second trimester of pregnancy, I invite my pregnant students to practice Deep Relaxation Pose on their left side. (For details, please see page 232 in chapter 9.)

Some people are uncomfortable with their eyes covered up. If this is the case, then create darkness by making a "hood" with a blanket over the head so there is nothing touching the face or eyes, but light is mostly blocked out.

PROPS NEEDED

There is just no getting around the fact that the most delicious Deep Relaxation Pose requires lots of props. But mostly you can use what you have already. It does help to have a yoga bolster, but most of the other props can be improvised.

- Nonslip yoga mat
- Five blankets if you have a bolster, otherwise seven
- Bolster
- Eye cover
- Yoga block
- Timer

Deep Relaxation Pose 1

BASIC

This is the classic pose. It does require a bit of a learning curve with the props. My suggestion is that if you are unfamiliar with the use of props that you begin slowly. Add the head support for a while and see how you like that. Then begin to add more props as makes sense for you. But always cover up, no matter what props you use or don't use, because it is impossible to relax if you are cold.

Add the next props in the following order: a prop under the knees, a roll under the ankles, and wrist support. If you add these props over time, not only will it help you learn about their placement, it will educate you on the effect of each prop as you gradually add them. Some students find that if they gather all their props and keep them in the place they practice, it is easier to practice Deep Relaxation Pose because the props are already in one place, just waiting for you.

Begin by spreading out your yoga mat. I like to put my mat on top of a plush area rug that covers part of the floor in my yoga room. I find I really like the extra padding the rug affords. Gather your props, including your timer.

Begin by folding all your blankets into Mountain Pose (this is what I call the main fold, because like Mountain Pose, it is "essential") as seen at the far right of figure 11.3. This shape is created by first folding the short ends of the blanket together, then folding the short ends together again, and finally, folding the remainder in half. This is the basic blanket shape that works well for all the setups in this chapter.

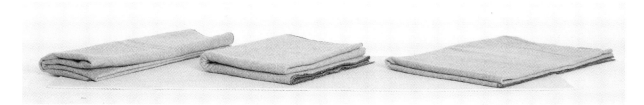

The sequence for folding the head blanket is as follows: First fold the blanket so that it is a bit uneven, or what I call "stair-stepped."

FIGURE 11.3

FIGURE 11.4

Next, lie on the tail or longer aspect of the blanket so that it supports the top of the scapulae. This means that the tail of the blanket goes under you a bit, a little past the C7–T1 spinal segments. To refresh your memory about the location of this area of your body, reach back and feel the "bump" at the end of your neck as the neck becomes trunk. It might help to find this area if you flex your neck a bit forward. You want the tail of the blanket to go a little past this, supporting the top third of the scapulae. Then the blanket is rolled slightly up, not under. This rolled-up part will support the C7–T1 vertebrae.

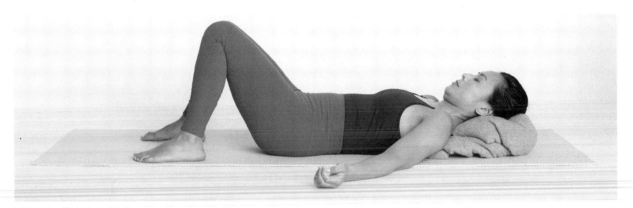

FIGURE 11.5   Place the bolster under your knees and the lower rolled blanket under your Achilles tendons. The knee support should support the knees about two times higher than the ankles are supported. If you are using a square bolster, use the block as shown. If you are using a round bolster, you do not need a block.

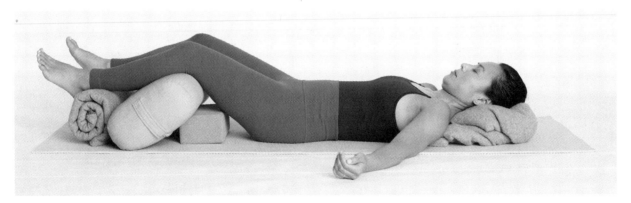

FIGURE 11.6   Now prepare the wrist support. This blanket fold is exactly the same as the one for neck and head support. Set your timer for twenty minutes, or for as long as thirty minutes if you wish. Now lie down. Put a blanket over you and remember to cover your eyes.

Take several minutes to make sure that you are totally comfortable. What might help this process is to feel if your arms and legs are feeling equidistant from your body. Most people feel more comfortable if their arms are

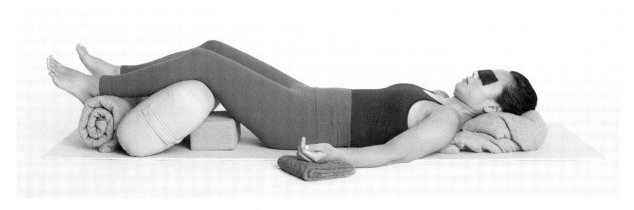

FIGURE 11.7

positioned wide out to the sides so the inner arm is not touching the trunk of their body. This wider position of the arms helps the scapulae lie flatter on the floor and facilitates easier breathing.

I like to begin Deep Relaxation Pose with some simple breathing. One of the easiest and most effective techniques is simply to slow your inhalations and exhalations and try to make them even. Inhale a normal amount, and then exhale a normal amount. For the next breath, make the inhalation a little longer and the exhalation to match it. But this time punctuate these long breaths with a shorter, normal breath. So the rhythm would be long slow inhalation, long slow exhalation, a normal breath in, a normal breath out. Then another long slow inhalation, long slow exhalation, normal breath in, normal breath out, and so on. If you feel any stress or find it difficult at the end of the exhalation, then merely shorten the long breaths, both in and out. This breathing rhythm should always feel easy and soothing. Try this rhythm for five to ten breaths and then let the breathing find its own intelligence once again and become soft, slow, light, and natural.

Release the arms and legs from the center of your trunk, like water flowing out and down from a mountain through the "rivers" of your arms, across a plain to the sea. Let the belly organs drop down into the pelvis with each exhalation. Soften the jaw, cheeks, and throat. Invite the eyelids to drop completely down, and release any tension you may hold in your scalp and around the back of your ears. Let your fingers curve naturally and easily toward your palm.

Now take your attention to the center of your brain. Enter the dark, cool, calm, and quiet center of your brain, as you would a vast temple or cathedral, and rest your attention lightly there. Just be. Let the air breathe you. Withdraw into your center. Receive the breath, receive the weight of the body, receive the moment. Give up ambition, give up movement, give up fear, and simply rest.

When your twenty-minute timer goes off, turn it off but continue to lie there for a couple of minutes more. Lightly begin to pay attention to your surroundings. Now inhale, and with an exhalation, bring your lower back ribs and back pelvic rim to the floor. Turn your legs internally so that your kneecaps are facing the ceiling. Continuing to hold your lower back down and your pelvis stable, gradually drag one heel toward you as your knee bends, and place one foot on the floor. Repeat for your other leg and roll to your side of choice.

I like to roll to the left; most students are told to roll to the right because "it is better for the heart." I have asked several doctors, including a couple of cardiologists about this idea and was told it was fine to roll to either side. Actually, the Indian medical science and art of Ayurveda recommends that lying on the left side can help with digestion.

Western medicine tells pregnant women to lie on the left side in the latter part of pregnancy to avoid impingement of blood vessels in the lower abdomen that bring blood to the placenta and thus the baby. But for most students, my suggestion is that you ask your body which side it "wants" to roll onto each time Deep Relaxation Pose is over, and then follow your body's wisdom by rolling to that side.

Lie on your side for at least thirty seconds to one minute. Make sure that your belly button is slightly facing the floor. Now use your arms to help you sit up. Let the chin drop to the chest as you come up. You are actually almost coming up back first. Sit until you feel oriented and ready before standing up and going on with your day.

Deep Relaxation Pose 2

LEGS ELEVATED

This variation of the basic Deep Relaxation Pose given above is done with the legs elevated and is especially enjoyable if you have been on your feet for hours working, cooking, or teaching yoga.

Begin by unrolling your mat and your props. You will need all your blankets stacked up or your bolster with some blankets added. You can also use an ottoman or take the seat cushion off your couch or use a yoga chair that has the seat covered by a blanket.

Fold the blanket for your head as was instructed in Deep Relaxation Pose 1 above. Place it and your eye cover near you. Now lie down and place your legs on your props. Make sure that the backs of your knees are supported and that your thighs are at an approximately 45° angle. Adjust your position, and when your legs feel supported and at ease, place your neck support under your head, tucking it firmly around your neck and shoulders, and make sure it supports your last cervical vertebrae, C7, and the first two thoracic vertebrae, T1 and T2. Add wrist support as instructed above.

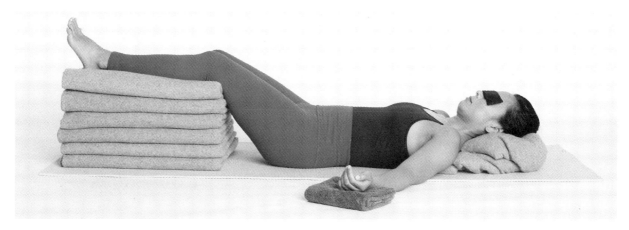

FIGURE 11.8

Set your timer for at least twenty minutes. Cover up with a blanket and place your eye cover over your eyes, being sure not to place weight on the eyes themselves.

Begin to let go. Let your back pelvis and sacrum sink into the floor. Invite your legs to let go of the actual and symbolic work that they have done all day to hold you up and help you walk.

Take a long slow inhalation and let it out slowly. Imagine all your belly organs are melting down onto the back of your pelvis. Release your fingers, cheeks, and the skin around your eyes. Imagine that your body is liquid and let it melt and spread over the floor.

Take a few deliberate breaths and then let go of changing your breath. In your imagination sink down below your breath; feel the movement associated with breath like the waves on the surface of the ocean. Rest deeply inside and allow this soft, light, surface movement of the body as you breathe almost imperceptibly. Retreat to the center of your brain and remain there with your consciousness.

When your timer goes off, quiet it, and continue to lie there and rest for a minute or so. Then bring your knees toward your chest and roll to the side. Begin to hear the sounds around you. Slowly sit up and enjoy the rest of your day.

Deep Relaxation Pose 3
WITHOUT PROPS

Once in a while a situation might arise when I really want to practice Deep Relaxation Pose but do not have any props. This variation is useful to have in your repertoire for those rare occasions. But I strongly suggest that as often as possible you do use props.

The one prop some people might need for "no prop" Deep Relaxation Pose is a blanket to support the head, neck, and shoulders. This might be necessary for those people who have a deep rib cage, that is, a rib cage that is deep from front to back. You will notice this if you or one of your students lies down on the back and the head hangs backward significantly so the chin is facing upward.

Sometimes this also happens to people who have a larger thoracic kyphosis. This means that the upper back rounds outward enough to cause the chest to be deeper and their head to hang backward when they lie down. If either of these is the case for you, use a blanket in this version of Deep Relaxation Pose to support your head, neck, and shoulders. Please refer to the instructions on how to fold and place the blanket in "Deep Relaxation Pose 1," above. Create the shape of the blanket you will need and then place it next to you. You will also want to have your eye cover near you to use once you are lying down.

To prepare, spread your yoga mat on a comfortable surface, either a rug or carpet for example. Set your timer now to about twenty-five to twenty-seven minutes; this will allow you time to set yourself up with a full twenty minutes of Deep Relaxation Pose time remaining.

Start by sitting with your legs stretched out in front of you. Notice your legs; make sure they are equidistant apart. Place your eye bag on one side of you where it will be within easy reach of your hand. Continue preparing by reaching down and pulling your calf muscles inward; this will allow your legs to roll out more comfortably.

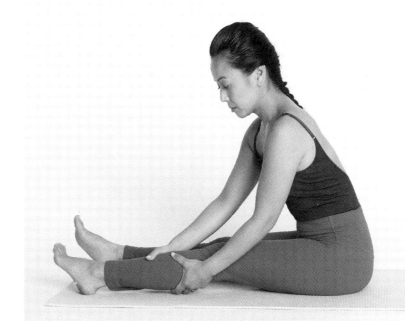

FIGURE 11.9

Next, pull the flesh of your upper thighs outward, the opposite direction in which you rolled your calves.

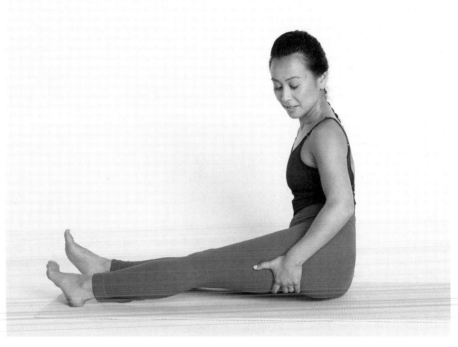

FIGURE 11.10

Now lean back on your forearms, and slide your thumbs under your body. Let your lower back round and begin to push with your forearms as if to move your body away from your feet. Do not actually move your body, but rather anchor your pelvis to the floor and stretch your back ribs away from it. Keep rounding your lower back.

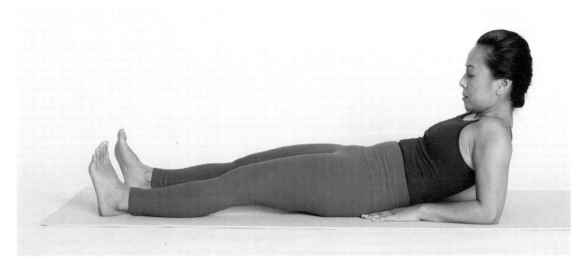

FIGURE 11.11   Gently place your back lower ribs on the floor and lie down. Notice how you are now resting on the middle of your sacrum and your back lower ribs, and that the lumbar spine has its natural curve, so it does not touch the floor.

Disturbing your shoulders as little as possible, hold your head and gently but firmly stretch out the back of your neck.

Now let your head down and place your skull on the flat place below your occipital ridge, which is prominent on the lower backside of your skull. Once the head is in place, put your eye cover on your breastbone using as little movement of your arm as possible. You will put it over your eyes in a moment.

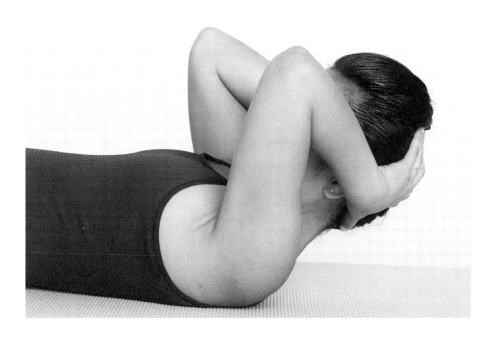

FIGURE 11.12

The next stage is to position the arms. Reach across your body with your right arm and take your left wrist. Pull your left arm firmly across your chest. It is very important that your left arm remains *totally* passive. Do not let your left arm "help" your right arm at all.

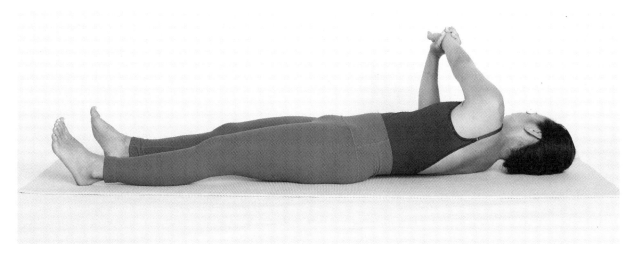

FIGURE 11.13

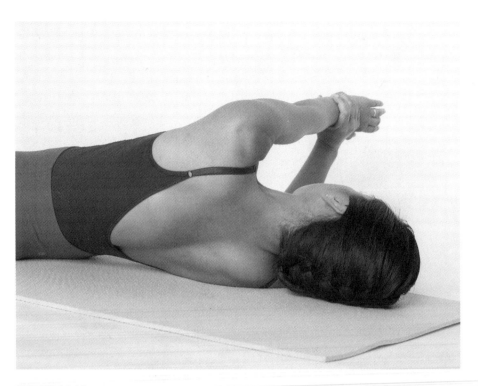

FIGURE 11.14

Not only are you pulling on your left arm, you are also letting your left scapula move with the arm, so the scapula moves toward the outer edge of your body.

Create as much space as you can between your vertebral column and your scapula. While still holding your left arm, place the left shoulder area on the floor so that the space between the scapula and the vertebral column is on the floor. Once your elbow is down, let your forearm almost fall to the floor and notice how much your left upper body lets go.

Put on your eye cover now using your right hand. Keeping the space you just created, and your left elbow on the floor, now place your right wrist in your left hand. Do not disturb the placement of your left scapula, your left upper arm, and your left elbow. Pull your right arm as we did the left, creating the space between the right scapula and the vertebral column as you did on the left, and once this space is created, then simply let your right arm flop to the floor. Do not let your arm down slowly. Rather, let it roll passively like a carpet unrolling with minimal control.

Finally, once again lift your head very slightly off the floor and drop your chin down, thus lengthening that space below your occipital ridge. Attempt to put that flat place on the floor. This will result in your chin remaining slightly lower than your forehead, which will facilitate a quieter brain.

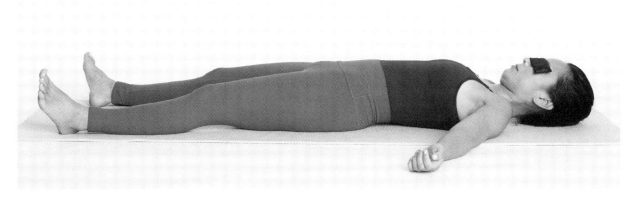

FIGURE 11.15

Notice the relationship of your bones with the floor. Feel your intimacy with the floor. Trust the floor to support you as you take several slow deep breaths. Invite your belly to let go. Coax your brain to drop backward toward the back of your skull. Allow your soft body to melt downward and flow outward. Enjoy the simplicity of this moment.

When your timer rings after twenty minutes, turn it off while disturbing yourself as little as possible. Once again take several long breaths. Now turn your kneecaps so that they look at the ceiling, and exhaling, bring your lower back and lower back ribs firmly to the floor. Hold this position while you drag one heel toward your buttocks as you bend the knee. Once you have completed this action, do the same with the other leg. Now roll onto your side of choice and lie there for at least a minute before using your arms to slowly bring you to a seated position. Take care to sit up slowly and notice how relaxed your body feels and how content your mind is. Enjoy this state as you move into your day.

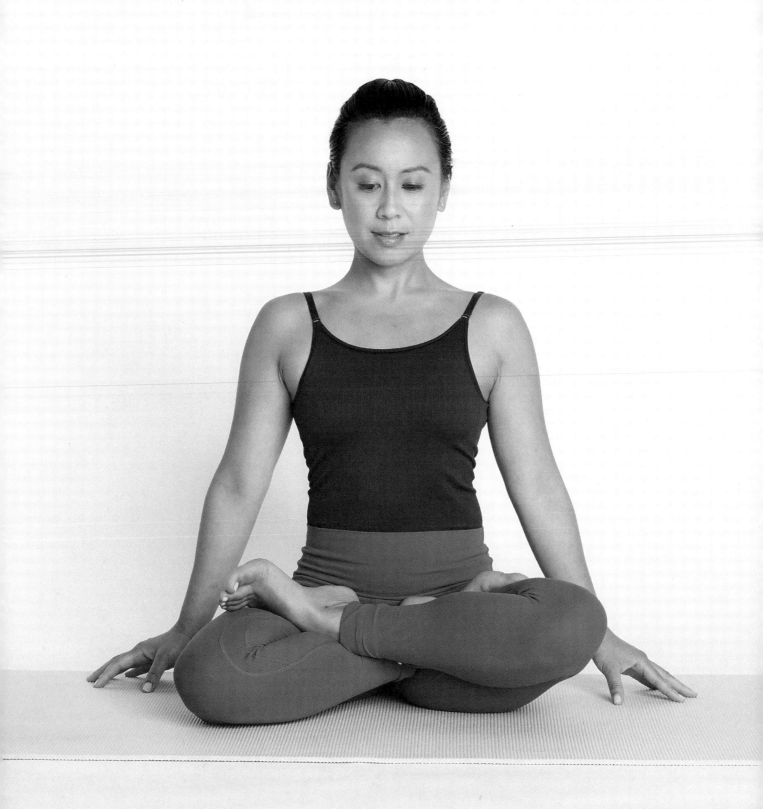

12

Questions and Answers

LEARNING MORE AND FEELING BETTER

Curiosity is essential for a life well lived.

WHILE THIS BOOK may have answered some of your questions about the practice of yoga asana, perhaps it has generated a few more. Here are some common questions and answers that you might like to explore.

Q: *Should I consult my doctor before I begin practicing yoga?*

A: Regular checkups are never a bad idea, and it is likewise a good idea to tell your doctor that you are taking up the practice of yoga asana.

Explain that you may be putting your head below your heart in standing forward bends and in mild inversions. Be sure to ask about any conditions or diagnoses you may have to hear her opinion on adding yoga asana to your health program.

Q: *What's the difference between a home practice and taking a class?*

A: Just like when one studies a musical instrument, for example, the lessons are there, in large part, to teach you how to practice. Taking regular yoga classes is something most people enjoy because it provides inspiration and a learning environment that keeps one safer and makes the poses more enjoyable.

But a home practice is necessary to actually help you integrate the learning you get from performing the poses on a deeper level into your body and your life. Students sometimes ask me if they should practice every day on their own. I always say, "Oh no, you don't need to practice every day, only on the days you want to feel better."

To guide you in creating a home practice, may I recommend my book *30 Essential Yoga Poses: For Beginning Students and Their Teachers*? It takes you through the basic poses in great detail, and there are also practice sequences at the back of the book that can be very helpful for developing a home practice.

Q: *Where can I find a qualified yoga teacher?*

A: One way is to check out the website YogaAlliance.org. This is an online listing service showing the location and training of thousands of teachers. Another way is to ask your friends if they know of a yoga teacher who is well trained.

You can also look around your neighborhood for a nearby yoga studio. But always take some time to find the right fit for you. Attend a class one time and see if you like the way that particular teacher teaches. There are many styles of asana practiced today, but your experience will be more satisfying if you find a style that is intuitively yours.

Notice during the class, not just what the teacher seems to know about her topic, but also, importantly, how she treats her students. Does she use respectful language when teaching the group and when she addresses you privately? Does she dress professionally? Does she ask permission to touch your body or just assume it is okay? Does she start and end her class on time? Does she regularly offer that oh-so-important fifteen to twenty minutes of relaxation at the end of class? Do you feel safe in her class? Does she challenge you to find your own limits in the pose, or does she push you to do more all the time? Is everyone in the class told to do exactly the same thing to the same degree? In other words, is she teaching people first and poses second?

Finally, just as there are many styles of asana practice, there are widely differing standards of training for yoga teachers. At this moment in time, there are no legal or professional requirements for being a yoga teacher in the United States. Anyone can call herself a yoga teacher and just start teaching. I highly recommend that you investigate the level of training your potential teacher has and how long her training lasted. Some training programs are as short as a weekend or two. I further suggest that you find a teacher who has been teaching at least two to five years, especially if you are a total beginner.

Q: *Where can I buy the props shown in this book?*

A: There are many online resources for buying yoga props; however, I prefer the props available from Hugger Mugger at huggermugger.com. This company is one of the very first suppliers of yoga props and has been in business for decades. I find their props beautiful, well made, and very useable. Additionally, I have always enjoyed my interactions with the staff. Most of the props used in this book are from Hugger Mugger. I recommend them highly.

Q: *When is the best time to practice?*

A: This is very individual. I find I prefer to practice first thing in the morning before I get involved with my day and before I eat anything. Maybe a cup of tea, and then to the mat. Otherwise if I wait too long after I get up in the morning to get on my mat, I often find myself pulled into other things, and the practice slips away.

However, the best time to practice is the time that practicing fits into your life. Maybe after the kids have gotten on the school bus, or midafternoon before they come home. Other people find they like to take a shower when arriving home from work, and then step onto the mat for a thirty-minute practice before dinner and evening activities. Find the time that most fits your life, and you will be more likely to practice regularly. Remember, these poses are almost magically able to shift your perspective, reduce your stress, and lessen, and even eliminate, those nagging everyday aches and pains. But remember: none of this can happen if you don't practice the poses.

Q: *How long after I eat should I wait to practice?*

A: While this varies widely, as you can imagine, do wait at least two hours after meals before getting on your mat. Most seasoned practitioners wait much longer.

Q: *How do I begin to integrate the principles presented in this book into my home practice?*

A: I would suggest beginning with one pose and integrating the new learning about that specific pose into your practice until it feels natural and easy for you. Then pick another pose to practice with, and so on. Taking time to integrate the new things you learn from this book into your body and mind will make things easier and more satisfying.

Q: *What is the best sequence for practicing the poses discussed in this book?*

A: One way is to follow the book chapter by chapter since the poses are sequenced in each chapter. Another way is to pick a class of poses like standing poses or seated ones, and focus on those for a while. Whatever you do, take time to enjoy your journey.

Q: *What if I am practicing something in class in the way that I learned from this book, and it feels good in my body, but my yoga teacher insists I do it another way? What should I do?*

A: One of the things I say most often when training teachers is "trust yourself first." Notice I did not say, "trust yourself only." Yoga is a very personal practice, whether you are practicing the ethical precepts, the poses, the breathing, or the meditation aspects.

If you are studying with someone you trust and respect, you will gradually be willing to let her teachings into your body and mind. But never give up your self-reflection, your own intuition, or your own feelings when you are in class.

Cultivate the awareness and courage to say if necessary, "No, thank you" to an adjustment or teaching suggestion because it doesn't feel right to you. This is how you will gain confidence in your own abilities to practice well.

Q: *Where did the yoga myths you discuss in the book, like tucking the tailbone in Mountain Pose, come from?*

A: I get asked that all the time. And I have a very unsatisfying answer to share with you. I don't really know. I recognize parts of these movement myths from what I learned in gym class, some I recognize as coming from dance classes I have taken, and some I observe being taught in fitness classes. Some of these myths seem just to be floating about the culture and are vaguely accepted as "true" principles for the moving body.

Q: *Where can I learn more about anatomy as it relates to teaching and practicing yoga asana?*

A: Together with my daughter, Lizzie Lasater, and my co-teacher, Mary Richards, we have created an online course called Experiential Anatomy. You can find out more about this course at www.lasater.yoga. This course was based on my book, *Yogabody: Anatomy, Kinesiology, and Asana*. Besides anatomy and movement principles, this book has a practice section at the end of each chapter.

I also teach workshops on this material, as does Mary Richards. Find me at www.judith.yoga and Mary Richards at www.maryrichardsyoga.com.

Q: *What about yoga philosophy? Is that an important part of the physical practice of asana?*

A: I found that my practice of yoga techniques was deepened when I began to study the wider philosophy of yoga. This helped me to put the techniques into a context that gave my practice more depth.

Check out www.judith.yoga for my online Yoga Philosophy class. It takes some of the main sutras and explains them in a way that is related to living and practicing yoga in today's world. You might also like another of my books titled *Living Your Yoga: Finding the Spiritual in Everyday Life*, which is about how to live the philosophy of yoga off the mat.

Notes

1.   Kyli Rodriguez-Cayro, "9 Ways Posture Affects Your Health That Might Surprise You," Bustle, April 18, 2018, www.bustle.com/p/9-ways-posture -affects-your-health-that-might-surprise-you-8793625.

2.   Esther Gokhale, *8 Steps to a Pain-Free Back: Natural Posture Solutions for Pain in the Back, Neck, Shoulder, Hip, Knee, and Foot* (Pendo Press, 2018), 21.

3.   A. I. Kapandji, *The Physiology of the Joints: The Spinal Column, Pelvic Girdle and Head* (Scotland: Handspring Publishing, 2019).

4.   Stacy Lu, "How Chronic Stress Is Harming Our DNA," *American Psychological Association* 45, no. 9 (October 2014): 28.

5.   Paul W. Hodges and Carolyn A. Richardson, "Contraction of the Abdominal Muscles Associated with Movement of the Lower Limb," *Physical Therapy* 77, no. 2 (1997): 132–42, discussion 142–4.

6.   Marc A. Russo, Danielle M. Santarelli, and Dean O'Rourke, "The Physiological Effects of Slow Breathing in the Healthy Human," *Breathe* 13, no. 4 (December 2017), https://breathe.ersjournals.com/content/13/4/298.

7.   Lu, "How Chronic Stress Is Harming Our DNA," 28.

Index

clavicle and, 81–82

in Deep Relaxation Poses, 226, 227, 234

in Downward-Facing Dog, 74, 87

holding firm, 83, 88–89

in Mountain Poses, 13, 16

natural movement of, 78–81, 83

shoulder joint and, 73

in Staff Pose, 90, 91

in Triangle Pose, 48–49

in Warrior I, 84

scapulohumeral rhythm. *See* glenohumeral rhythm

scapulothoracic joint. *See* scapulae (shoulder blades)

scoliosis, 4

screw home mechanism, 102

Seated Forward Bend (Paschimottanasana), 41, 42–44, 173

Seated Twist (Marichyasana III), 68–69

self-awareness, 3, 161, 201

self-knowledge, 3, 168

semimembranosus muscle and tendon, 98

serratus

anterior, 78

posterior, 197–98

Setu Bandhasana. *See* Bridge Pose

shoulder blades. *See* scapulae (shoulder blades)

shoulder joint, 27, 73, 75–77

in Elbow Stand, 159

flexion and abduction of, 78, 81–82

in Handstand, 155–56

holding still, 83

in Mountain Poses, 16

natural movement of, 74

stability in, 186

in Warrior I, 84

See also glenohumeral joint

Shoulder Stand (Sarvangasana), 19, 132, 133, 134, 165

apana in, 174

cautions for, 20, 21, 145

cervical spine in, 25–26

See also Supported Shoulder Stand (Salamba Sarvangasana)

shoulder width, 153

Side Plank Pose (Vasisthasana), 126–27

Side-Lying Deep Relaxation Pose, 178, 223, 224

silence, 14, 186, 207, 213, 221, 222

sitting

in breathing awareness practices, 203

jalandhara bandha and, 28

Mountain Pose, 16

pelvis in, 38

prevalence of, 3, 8

sacrum in, 46, 62–63

well, 7

sitting bones. *See* ischial tuberosities (sitting bones)

sit-ups, 113, 121

sleep, 132, 179, 199, 213, 215, 216, 220

soft tissue, 27

imbalances in, 106

in joints, 26, 47

pain in, 7

stressing, 5, 6, 25, 45, 64, 94

See also fascia (connective tissue); ligaments; tendons

stability, 103, 143

abdominal muscles in, 114–16, 118–21, 122

in Elbow Stand, 139–40

in knees, 94, 99, 102, 103–4

in Mountain Pose, 11, 13

in Plank Pose, 88

sacroiliac joint and, 47, 59, 60, 61, 63–64, 65

of shoulder joint, 83

spinal curves in maintaining, 4–5, 9, 10

Staff Pose (Dandasana), 97–98

Standing Forward Bend (Uttanasana), 133, 134

hip joint in, 40–42

instructions, 146–50

resting in, 157

standing/standing postures, 1, 40–41

apana and prana in, 172

inversion in, 133

knees in, 96, 98, 102

in neutral, ascertaining, 8–9

pelvis in, 38, 47

sacroiliac joint in, 61, 63

sternum (breastbone), 75, 76, 116, 196

in forward bends, 71, 87

in jalandhara bandha, 28

in Mountain Pose, 14

Vasisthasana. *See* Side Plank Pose

vena cava syndrome, inferior, 177–78

vertebrae
    cervical, 7, 20, 21, 22, 26, 85, 187, 229
    lumbar, 21, 40, 196, 197, 203
    spinal curves and, 3, 5, 6, 9
    thoracic, 3, 26, 132, 229

vertebral column, 2–5
    abdominal muscles and, 114, 115, 120
    anterior longitudinal ligament of, 59
    curves of, 1–2, 16, 147, 203, 217
    diaphragm and, 196
    distorting, 6–7, 8–9
    flexion and extension of, 16–17
    in forward bends, 40, 150
    in lying down, 218, 234
    and pelvis, relationship between, 37–38, 42, 46, 47
    in Plank Pose 1, 125
    during pregnancy, 177
    sympathetic curves of, 10, 16–17, 146

Viparita Karani. *See* Legs-Up-the-Wall Pose

Virabhadrasana. *See* Warrior

Vrksasana. *See* Tree Pose

Warrior (Virabhadrasana)
    Warrior I, 84–85
    Warrior II, 50, 81
    Warrior III, 103

whiplash, 29, 32, 145, 181

Wide-Angle Seated Forward Bend (Upavistha Konasana), 57, 64, 98

Wide-Legged Forward Bend (Prasarita Padotta-nasana), 133, 134, 151–52

withdrawal, conscious mental (*pratyahara*), 192

wrists, 134–35, 136–38

xiphoid process, 116, 117, 118, 196

yoga myths
    on blood oxygen, 199
    on breathing, 200, 211
    on Deep Relaxation Pose, 214, 220, 221
    on inversions, 132, 144
    on knees, 106
    on neck, 20, 219
    origins of, 240
    on pranayama, 193
    on shoulder joints, 74
    on spine and pelvis, relationship of, 38
    on tucking tailbone, 55, 61
    on women, practicing as, 168, 170, 171, 172, 174, 179

yoga practice
    being one's Self in, 2
    best time for, 239
    breathing in, 193–94
    eating and, 202, 239
    integrating new principles into, 239
    studio and home practice, differences between, 237–38
    in West, 168
    yoga philosophy and, 241
    See also asana; Restorative yoga

Yoga Sutras of Patanjali, 27, 192, 193

Yogabody, 240–41

About the Author

Judith Hanson Lasater, PhD, PT, C-IAYT, E-RYT-500, YACEP®, has taught yoga around the world since 1971. She is a founder of the Iyengar Yoga Institute in San Francisco, California, as well as the *Yoga Journal* magazine, which is published in a number of countries. Ms. Lasater frequently trains teachers in virtually every state of the union and is often an invited guest at international yoga conventions. She is president emeritus of the California Yoga Teachers Association as well as the author of numerous articles on yoga and health for nationally recognized magazines.

She was featured in *Self* magazine in 1998 as one of the outstanding yoga teachers in the US. In 2000, she was selected by *Yoga Journal* as one of the outstanding yoga teachers shaping yoga practice in America today. She was selected by *Natural Health* magazine, on the occasion of their fortieth anniversary, as one of the five people in the US who has had the most influence on natural health in America during those forty years. In 2015, *Yoga Journal* selected her as "Editor's Choice" for the most influential yoga teacher in the US in the last forty years.

She is the author of nine books, including: *Restore and Rebalance: Yoga for Deep Relaxation* (2017), *What We Say Matters: Practicing Nonviolent Communication* (2009), *YogaBody: Anatomy, Kinesiology, and Asana* (2009), *A Year of Living Your Yoga: Daily Practices to Shape Your Life* (2006), *Yoga Abs: Moving from Your Core* (2005), *Yoga for Pregnancy: What Every Mom-to-Be Needs to Know* (2004), *30 Essential Yoga Poses: For Beginning Students and Their Teachers* (2003), *Relax and Renew: Restful Yoga for Stressful Times* (2005), and *Living Your Yoga: Finding the Spiritual in Everyday Life* (2000).